Jane Scrivner's

WATER
DETOX

514-240-6549

Other Books by Jane Scrivner

Detox Yourself
Detox Your Mind
Detox Your Life
The Little Book of Detox
Total Detox
The Quick-Fix Hangover Detox
Stay Young Detox
LaStone Therapy

Jane Scrivner's

WATER DETOX

Total Health and Beauty in 8 Easy Steps

PIATKUS

Visit the Piatkus website!

Piatkus publishes a wide range of best-selling fiction and non-fiction, including books on health, mind, body & spirit, sex, self-help, cookery, biography and the paranormal.

If you want to:
- read descriptions of our popular titles
- buy our books over the Internet
- take advantage of our special offers
- enter our monthly competition
- learn more about your favourite Piatkus authors

VISIT OUR WEBSITE AT: www.piatkus.co.uk

Copyright © 2002 Jane Scrivner

First published in 2002 by
Piatkus Books Limited
5 Windmill Street
London W1T 2JA
e-mail: info@piatkus.co.uk

This edition published in 2004

The moral rights of the author have been asserted

A catalogue record for this book is available from the British Library

ISBN 0 7499 2492 6

Edited by Barbara Kiser
Design by Paul Saunders

This book has been printed on paper manufactured with respect for the environment using wood from managed sustainable resources

Typeset by Phoenix Photosetting, Chatham, Kent
Printed in Denmark by Nørhaven Paperback A/s Viborg

This one's for Kevin. May we follow this programme, hydrate, and grow old and healthy together. With my love, Jane.

Contents

Introduction   1

1. Water for Life   10

2. The 18-Day H$_2$O Nutrition Programme   41

3. Hydrotherapy   75

4. Thalassotherapy   98

5. Watercise   109

6. Youth Dew   116

7. Healing Waters   138

8. Go with the Flow   147

Further Reading   194

Useful Addresses   196

Index   199

Introduction

LOADS OF ENERGY, GLOWING SKIN, great health, vitality, bright eyes, no aching joints, no grumbling illnesses, total motivation and a body to die for ... by just drinking the right amount of water? The Water Detox will prove to you that water is really and truly all you need to feel like this.

By following a programme of drinking, bathing, cleansing and exercising with the aid of water, all this can be yours in just 18 days or less. You will feel the benefits after just a few days and they can last for the rest of your life.

Something we take for granted can grant us everything we have wanted. Simply pour a glass and feel the goodness flow.

Water, air and food are the three things essential for life. We know we would die without air and we know we have to eat every day to survive, but we still ignore the need for water. We simply don't drink enough water, no matter how many times we are told. Well, it's time to listen ...

Total hydration is total health. Our bodies are 75 per cent water. If we drop this by just 2 per cent, we are dehydrated. As soon as we are dehydrated our bodily functions slow down and we begin to operate inefficiently.

How many of these feel familiar to you?

- Tiredness
- Bad circulation
- High blood pressure
- Headaches
- Dizziness
- Aching joints
- Dry and wrinkled skin
- Back pain
- Urinary infections
- Slow metabolism
- Low immunity
- Build-up of toxins
- Cellulite
- Slow thought processes
- Stress
- Weight gain
- Indigestion.

These are all caused by dehydration – not chronic dehydration, just simple day-to-day dehydration. Although it seems extraordinary, you can even die from this.

If you have any of these symptoms or maybe all of them, it may just be that bringing your consumption of water up to 2 litres every day can change your life. There is no danger in drinking water correctly. It is relatively inexpensive, it is readily available and the benefits are truly phenomenal.

The Water Detox will flush out your body and your life. It will cleanse and rinse away problems from the small and irritable to the huge, life-changing kind. Just as water feeds and nourishes, it will also water the seeds of change and help still the swell of stress and anxiety. Water can affect anything and everything. Following the Water Detox will have the same profound effect on you, and your future.

Not only does drinking the stuff hugely improve our quality of life; being near it, getting in it or playing on it can have some phenomenal effects too. You have nothing to lose and so much to gain. Try the programme for 18 days and see how you can change the rest of your life.

Water is something that we never give a second's thought to. We never consider the water freely running and being wasted from our tap when we wash our hands or clean our teeth, but the water we waste could be enough to mean the difference between life and death to someone living in a country with drought conditions. You never know what you have until it is gone.

Water is all around us, within us, in the air we breathe, in our skin cells, organs, and blood. We lose water all the time, when we sweat, talk and breathe. We need to replace water all the time to stay fully hydrated. Water is an essential nutrient – it truly is the elixir of life. Nothing is as important to life and nothing is so undervalued.

If we take water away, then we take away the essence of life.

THE 18-DAY PROGRAMME

Over the next 18 days you will follow a programme that will introduce water into each and every aspect of your life. We will introduce it slowly so that your body can start to use the water rather than just deal with it.

We will teach you how to drink. It may sound easy, but the reason most people give up drinking such relatively large amounts of water is because they go from nothing to the full 2 litres overnight. Not only is this very difficult for the body to assimilate, but it is also the most ineffective way you can make the change. The side effects of 'drowning' your body with so much water will almost certainly put you off. If you get it right from the beginning, you are more likely to stick to the habit and then it will become a totally natural – in fact, essential – part of your life.

The 18-day programme contains an 8-point plan. Just as water flows continuously, so does the programme. Once you have learnt how to drink water and to appreciate water as described in the first point, then you can start wherever you want to and follow the flow. Get water running freely through your body, and feel the effects.

1. Water for Life

Water for life takes us through types of water, ways to drink water, ways to appreciate water and a small taste of what our lives would be like without water. Water for life looks at the way water behaves and how it can totally balance because it knows no alternative. It is a great leveller because it always finds its own level.

2. The 18-Day H$_2$O Nutrition Programme

A programme to nourish and water your body, including foods that contain at least 50 per cent water and feed your body with the essential fluids and nutrients it needs. We will be drinking 2 litres but we will also expect to get about another litre through our newfound water diet. You will be surprised how much water you can get from food and how you shouldn't get thirsty while eating if your foods contain enough water.

There are recipes and meal ideas as well as an indication of how to cook your foods to preserve their water content and not drain it. You won't be on a diet but you will be following a strict nutritional programme. Weight loss will come naturally as we cleanse and feed our bodies. Seventy-five per cent of our hunger pangs are actually signals of thirst – our body's call for water.

3. Hydrotherapy

Water as therapy. Water is one of the most therapeutic elements we have in our lives. In moments of stress, the first thing we do is have a bath. We forget that the bath contains water. It is not the bathroom that does the trick, and it is not the lighting of the candles – it is actually the way we surround our bodies with water, hot or cold, that will do the trick. The resonance and vibration of the water is the balancing element. Sitting in an empty bath, lighting the candles, shutting the door and pumping up the heating will do nothing. Add the water and you are transformed. We forget that water is the thing; we have taken it for granted but from this part forward it will be recognised and valued for all the things it can do for us. It is relatively inexpensive and it's on tap. Use it.

You will be introducing new ways to enjoy water.

4. Thalassotherapy

Using the power of the sea to transform. The nutritional content of the sea, its therapeutic qualities and calming nature, all combine to bring the excitement of the oceans into your life and your bathroom. The sea supports and maintains a life force and is powerful and mysterious. When you absorb a little bit of this power and mystery, the world will truly be your oyster, with you as the pearl on centre stage.

5. Watercise

Exercise in water becomes effortless. Water removes the impact, the jolts and the strains. Exercise can be any sport; it doesn't have to be just exercise. As a way to increase the heart rate and improve fitness and vitality, water is wonderful. Water adds resistance and effort but it doesn't damage. We will address ways to keep the body toned and fit by looking at ways to introduce watercise into your life. No more gym kits, just fabulous swimming gear to double up by the pool or beach towel. Forget trainers, just get in the swim and see your body transform and become svelte and slim, toned and trimmed.

6. Youth Dew

Water and hydration to make your body glow with health and vitality. Adding water to your current routine will boost and improve your skin. Adding water to a non-existent routine will show you just how effective and important taking care of number one can be. In just a few days you will see your complexion change, look fresher and younger, and all with the cheapest skin care product available – yes, water. With varying uses of hot and cold water you will see that keeping the body fully hydrated both internally and externally will transform it and get people really thinking about your age and level of fitness – 'She looks fabulous', 'What is his secret', 'I don't know how she does it.' Water is the best-kept beauty secret, and also the worst kept, because it is all around us, but unless we use it we have wasted the opportunity to look and feel beautiful, naturally.

7. Healing Waters

Having an understanding of how water affects the body will give you a true picture of just how it can nurture and mend us. If we are made of the stuff, we need to know what it can do for and to us. We can starve ourselves if we become dehydrated, but we can nourish every cell if we know just what it does. Water should become our 'first port of call' if we feel even the slightest bit out of sorts. Water will be your medicine for the next 18 days: feel the difference, feel your energy levels increase and feel your mind fill with fast-flowing thoughts and ideas.

8. Go with the Flow

Water has energy, vibration and resonance. It can be full of vigour or calm, and change form, state or direction. It can be made to hold a 'memory' of other substances, and it can wipe everything away and start with a clean slate.

The moon and sun control the flow of tides and water, and we can begin to see that we, too, are affected much as the tides are. We ebb and flow, are high and low – exactly the same as water. Learning the way water behaves will give us some insight into just how much we change with the same influences. Becoming aware of this change and adding it to our lives allows us to explore many more strengths and possibilities for change than we ever considered before.

We can cleanse negative flow from our lives by practising the Chinese art of Feng Shui, and understand the vibrational powers by looking at homeopathy and flower essences – elixirs of life that use the simple and complicated aspects of water for healing.

Where you are striking a stress-free balance or looking for dramatic change, once you have harnessed the power of water you will be able to use it to your best advantage.

Each section will take you through the steps you can try. Each section will introduce many new ideas but you will only be asked to take up a few of them. You can do more, but the programme is designed to get you into the 'habit' of water so that you will take to it like the proverbial duck. There is a checklist to make sure that you are doing everything you need to. If you want to add to this, then go ahead; but if you want to follow it to the letter, this will show you the beauty of water, the phenomenal effects it will have on your life and the taste it will give you for more. Go on: dip your toe …

USING THE PROGRAMME

1. Value Your Water

Start the programme with a water appreciation exercise. Spend a day seeing how much you take it for granted, yet how wonderful it is.

2. Cleanse Internally

Start the 18-Day H_2O Nutrition Programme.

3. Harness Your Personal Healing Flow

Keep your own Moon Diary and monitor yourself; get your water to work for you and take your own personal elixirs for life.

4. Refresh and Rejuvenate Your Life

Use water in your home and your life to cleanse.

5. Tone Your Body and Banish Cellulite

Have three hydrotherapy and three thalassotherapy treatments during the 18 days.

6. Achieve Beautiful Skin

Introduce your hydrating skin care plan for the full 18-day period.

7. Revitalise Your Body

Exercise with, in or on water.

8. Healing Waters

Learn about how to use water as first aid, literally.

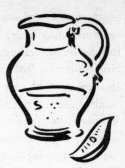

The Checklist

To make sure that you do not leave out any aspect of your Water Detox, copy this list and stick it to your noticeboard or fridge door. Refer to it daily to check that you are getting the best out of the programme and that you are feeling totally hydrated.

- I started the programme with my water appreciation experience.

- I have drunk 2 litres of pure water today.

- I have eaten 3 large or 5 smaller meals made up of foods from the food lists in the book.

- I am planning to have 3 thalassotherapy treatments during my programme.

- I am planning 3 hydrotherapy treatments during my programme.

- I have followed the skin care routine for body and face today and every day.

- I am planning to exercise in, by or on water every other day of the programme.

- I am checking in with my body each day to see how water can improve my health.

- I am keeping my Moon Diary every day.

- I am checking the water around me to create flow and wealth.

Using this template for the next 18 days will ensure that you are achieving flow in every aspect of your life. Water will seep quietly into your life, rehydrating you and plumping up your health and vitality.

1

Water for Life

EVEN THOUGH IT IS EASILY got in most of the world, and known to be good for us ... and despite it being cheaper than anything else we drink and being 'on tap' in every Western home, we clearly still don't get it where the importance of water consumption is concerned.

Here is a list of the most basic facts. It truly is amazing that we can get it so wrong when drinking enough water is really so simple, and more effective at enhancing wellbeing than almost anything else in our lives except for the air we breathe. Read on, and hopefully you will be persuaded to pour yourself your first glass to recovery.

- The brain is 75 per cent water.

- Blood is 92 per cent water.

- Bones are 22 per cent water.

- Muscles are 75 per cent water.

- Brain cells are 82 per cent water.

- Moderate dehydration can cause headaches and even dizziness.

- The brain weighs 1.5 kilogrammes, of which 200 grammes are actual brain – the rest is water.

- We need water to exhale.

- Water inside the body regulates our body temperature.

- Water helps us to breathe as it moistens air on inhalation.

- Water helps remove toxins and waste.

- On hot days, sweating causes us to lose up to 16 glasses of water per day.

- 2 out of 3 people drink the recommended minimum of 8 glasses of water a day.

- Thirst indicates a state of dehydration.

- Not drinking enough water can result in dry and itchy skin, feelings of lethargy upon waking, and tiredness during the day.

- Long-term dehydration causes high blood pressure, bad circulation, bad digestion, poor kidney function and slow bodily operation and processing.

- We lose as much water when we are sleeping as we do when we are awake.

- The body needs almost as much water in cold weather as it does in hot.

- Approximately 90 per cent of the world's population is chronically dehydrated.

- We are so used to feelings of thirst that we mistake them for hunger.

- Mild dehydration slows down metabolism by as much as 3 per cent.

- Lack of water is the number one cause of tiredness.

- Just 8 to 10 glasses of water a day could ease up to 80 per cent of general aches and pains.

- It only takes a 2 per cent drop in hydration to slow down recall, give trouble with basic maths, and cause difficulty in focusing on reading or screen work.

- 5 glasses of water per day decrease the risk of colon cancer by 45 per cent.

- 5 glasses of water a day cut the risk of breast cancer by 79 per cent.

- 5 glasses of water a day reduce the risk of bladder cancer by 50 per cent.

Now pour yourself a glass and feel your body say 'Thank you.'

Here are some further facts about how water is an indispensable part of our lives:

- 97 per cent of the water on our planet is in the oceans.

- The Atlantic, Arctic, Antarctic, Indian and Pacific Oceans cover 75 per cent of the earth with water.

- 2 per cent of the earth's water is ice.

- 0.8 per cent of our water comes from the ground.

- 0.2 per cent of our water is in rivers, lakes, clouds and springs.

Only 1 per cent of the earth's water is available for human use

- 75 per cent of the water we use is used in the bathroom.

- Leaving the tap on while we clean our teeth uses up to 91 litres of water.

- Toilets use between 16 and 23 litres of water per flush.

- Washing machines use about 190 litres per cycle.

- Dishwashers use approximately 65 litres per cycle.

Water and Human Survival

The human body contains over 75 per cent water. Water is the body's transport system, which moves nutrients around it as well as carrying waste out of it. Water breaks down food, keeps your body temperature balanced and your skin elastic. We can live for weeks without food but only a few days without water.

Water on Our Planet

As we've seen, 97 per cent of all the water on our planet is in the oceans. The Atlantic, Arctic, Antarctic, Indian and Pacific Oceans cover about three-quarters of the earth with water. About 2 per cent of the earth's water is ice, while 0.8 per cent of water is groundwater and less than 0.2 per cent makes up rivers, lakes, clouds, and springs.

Water Usage

Why is so little of the earth's water available for human use? Since 97 per cent of the earth's water is saltwater, and can only be used if processed by desalination plants, and over 2 per cent is polluted or part of the ice cap, less than 1 per cent of all water is actually available for human use. In the home, three-quarters of all water is used in the bathroom. Letting the water run while brushing your teeth can increase daily usage by up to 91 litres. Older toilets use up to 23 litres of water per flush (low flow use 16 litres). During California's drought of 1989 many restaurants stopped serving water to their customers unless they requested it. It was considered better to have a dirty car and a brown lawn than to waste water. Bottled water became a necessary alternative to tap water because as the reservoirs got lower, the concentration of minerals and chemicals in tap water increased and the taste deteriorated.

WHAT IS WATER?

Water is something we take far too much for granted. We live by it, we are born from it and we survive on it. But we rarely think about what it really is. Here are a few of its forms and qualities:

- It is natural.

- It is a solid, a liquid, a vapour.

- It can be floated on and it can be travelled under.

- It has a skin, and we can be physically supported by it.

- It dissolves almost everything else we come into contact with except oil.

- It is snow, ice, clouds, rain and hailstones.

- It is sea, ocean, lake, pool and pond.

- It can be seen in the morning as dew and early morning mists that fade to show a wonderful day.

- It flows over waterfalls and it runs in underground streams.

- We need it to survive.

- If we don't respect it, it can cause death and destruction.

- It generates power.

- It trickles and giggles.

- It washes away everything, physical and emotional.

So far, so good. But what is water, in and of itself?

Put very, very simply, water is a chemical compound made of two types of atom, one atom of oxygen and two of hydrogen. That is why we see water written as H_2O.

In chemistry, atoms or molecules are either negatively or positively charged. Both hydrogen and oxygen are negatively charged so they actually 'repel' each other. They spend their time trying to get away from each other. This is one of the reasons why water is flexible and can change form so easily. If you pour a jug of water over a table surface, it spreads absolutely everywhere and if you collect this same water into a jug and freeze it, it becomes a solid very quickly. Add salt and it boils at a higher temperature, and add it to a thickening product such as gravy granules and it will expand to form a thick sauce. It is one of the most flexible things we have.

An extremely important aspect of the Water Detox is the effect water can have on us at any level. If you think of the flexibility of water, and then consider that we are 75 per cent water, then you can see that it must also effect some fairly major changes within us, both physically and mentally.

Water's electrical charge does more than make it flexible. Along with water, absolutely every other organism, cell or atom on this earth also has an electrical charge. So water is affected by every person, every body, every item, every energy field, idea or emotion that it comes into contact with.

Water has its own electrical vibration and resonance. And if you put water next to anything else, it will respond to that object's vibration or resonance in some way or another. This is more specifically covered in 'The Memory of Water' (see page 151), but it is worth lodging in the mind the fact that we can alter the state of water ourselves, and water can also alter our own state. As we are electromagnetically charged, and are 75 per cent water, water will have profound effects on us – every single time.

Our response can be minuscule or huge, 'slow-drip' and almost imperceptible, or immediate, even fatal. Water has the ability to cure and to promote harmony and homeostasis (healthy balance).

In fact, the list of things water can do is amazing:

• It can generate power and electricity by harnessing wave energy.

• It can help plants grow for food to feed a nation or the world.

• It can carry goods from one side of the world to another.

• It can give life to the marine world.

- It can rehydrate a sick, dehydrated body.

- It can wash stubborn marks from our clothes.

- It can wash a coastline away.

- It can force its way through land to create riverbeds.

- It is the basis for nearly every meal we eat.

- It can relax us and keep us sane.

- It can warm us and protect us.

- It can preserve things for long periods of time.

- It can dilute almost all substances so much that they are hardly there.

Water really can do anything. But we still don't give it a second thought, unless we don't have it. Then it becomes an obsession, or a cause, or a dangerous and potentially fatal situation. Something so important is incredibly undervalued. The Water Detox programme will give you endless reasons or even just one that will make it the most important thing in your life. And all you need to do is turn on the tap.

WATER APPRECIATION

The easiest and most straightforward way to appreciate water is to take it away. This can be very difficult, and is also potentially unhealthy. The next best thing is to make sure you are aware of and appreciate water every time you use it.

On the first day of the programme, enjoy water and indulge with water so that you can see how difficult life would be without it. Really try to imagine what a waterless day would be like. You will be amazed at how much we take water for granted. This exercise will bring home to you the importance of water in just a few short hours, and hopefully make you treasure and preserve it from this point forward.

You don't know what you have until it is gone.

Of course, we cannot take water out of our lives totally. It is all around us and it is everywhere. We cannot cancel the sea or put a stop on the rivers, and we certainly cannot control the weather or the skies, but we can stop turning on the tap or driving the car without taking the time to appreciate how important water is.

The day will start from the moment you wake up. Once you become aware of how you use water, you will begin to see that it is also an incredibly important social tool.

Start the Day Upon Rising

Take a wonderfully refreshing shower of warm water. Feel the water run over your body and cleanse away the drowsiness of the night before. Once your body is wet, get out of the shower and stand on a bath mat. Use an exfoliating scrub with eucalyptus and peppermint essential oils to slough away the dead skin cells and refresh the skin. Climb back into the shower and rinse away. Once again, feel the water cleanse your body and stand there for a few extra minutes. Something you take for granted every day should now be totally experienced and appreciated. How would it feel to start the day without being able to wash this way, without a shower, scrub, or even a wash ... ? You can just get up and get dressed.

After you have dried off and got dressed, proceed through your day thinking about the water you use. Every time you turn on the tap, consider how you would do the job if the tap was dry. Go through your day working out how you would be able to do everyday, normal jobs without the use of water. You could not:

• Drink water – with ultimately fatal consequences.

• Wash, bathe or shower.

• Wash your hair.

• Use styling appliances that use steam.

• Clean your teeth.

• Take pills or medicines with a glass of water, or mix water into foods.

17

- Put the heating on – the system uses water in the radiators.

- Boil the kettle.

- Drive your car, as the engine is water-cooled.

- Go out in the rain unless totally waterproofed so that no water touches you.

- Do the washing up.

- Put the dishwasher on.

- Do the laundry.

- Iron unless you turn the steam setting to off.

- Clean the house, as household cleaners contain water.

- Make a cup of tea.

- Go to a coffee morning.

- Take the children to the pool.

- Water your garden or houseplants.

- Bake.

- Drink anything in a meeting.

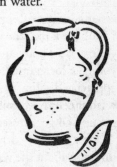

- Go for a walk anywhere where you can see water, sea, river, lake, pond, or brook. There would be no waterfalls, fountains or other water features in your conservatory.

- Cook anything that requires water as an ingredient, or as a cooking medium.

- Microwave anything that needs water added to steam it.

- Wash your hands.

- Have beauty treatments that use water to mix the product or use it to cleanse the body.

- Play in the snow in the winter.

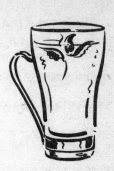

- Go ice skating.

- Soak anything.

- Swim or do any aqua aerobics.

- Sweat – it uses your bodily fluids.

- Have a glass of wine or beer.

- Have a relaxing bath at the end of the day.

- Take a glass of water to bed with you.

- Sleep soundly because your body is dehydrated.

And if you thought about all the ways you take water for granted then here are some you probably missed out:

- You were still breathing, and it takes water to do that.

- Your blood was still circulating through your body, and it takes water to do that.

- Your cells were still growing within your body and exchanging fluid from one side to another.

- Your sweat glands were still producing sweat.

- Your spinal discs were still supporting your spinal column.

- Your joints were still cushioned at every move by water.

- Your lungs were still exchanging fluids as you breathed.

- Your kidneys were still flushing through.

- Your body was still functioning.

- Your plumbing was still working at home.

- Your drains were still flushing water away.

- The sewer system was still protecting you from waste and flooding if it was raining.

You see, even if you try to appreciate water, there are still many, many ways we take it for granted and don't fully appreciate it.

To end your water appreciation day, you should take the time to truly appreciate water.

The Water Detox Bath

You will need:
Sunflower oil
Rose essential oil
Orange essential oil
Ylang ylang essential oil
Lavender essential oil

Pour 1 dessertspoon of sunflower oil into a bowl. Into this put 3 drops each of the above essential oils. Close the bathroom windows and door. Run a warm bath and gently pour in the oil blend. Stir the water with your hand 9 times in the figure 8. This will thoroughly mix the blend into the water. Let the water go still. Light a large candle at the end of the bath, preferably on a shelf or window ledge, somewhere you can see it when you are relaxing in the bath. Turn the lights down or even off and get into the bath.

As you relax into the water start to be aware of how the water feels against your skin. See how it supports your body and runs between your fingers and toes. Rub the oily blend from the surface of the water over your skin and see the droplets of the oil and water separate and fall. Take deep breaths in through your nose and smell the fragrance as it enters your mind and body. Stay in the water and feel how it relaxes your body and calms you. See how it makes you feel good just being surrounded by fresh, warm water. Imagine that this is the last bath you will ever be able to take, that this is the last time you can ever cleanse in this way. Appreciate how wonderful and versatile water is.

As you leave the bath, pat dry your body and moisturise your skin with your favourite body cream. Wrap up warm and either relax for an hour or go to bed and have sweet dreams . . .

How to drink water

Now that you are more aware of how water affects us, it is time to start using it to your best advantage – not to waste it but to use it to improve your quality of life and health.

Drinking the correct amounts of water can make phenomenal differences to our bodies and our lives. You will soon notice incredible levels of energy, glowing skin, weight loss, reduction of cellulite, better immunity, less fatigue and lethargy, the ability to think straight throughout the day and a general, all-round increased level of health and wellbeing.

Simply going from no water intake, unless heavily disguised in tea, coffee or alcohol, to 2 litres per day on a regular basis may just be a shock to the system if not done correctly.

If done correctly, it should only take your body 2 or 3 days to get used to the extra water you begin to use as part of everyday cleansing. Initially, it is likely and totally normal that you will feel as if you are spending your life on your way to or from the bathroom. So don't start to drink the right amount of water if you know you have a 3-hour examination to sit. Once the first few days have passed you will wonder how you ever survived.

There are a few simple rules to follow in order to get the best results and immediate effects:

- Drink at least 2 litres of water per day.

- On a hot day or in the summer, increase the daily amount by at least half a litre.

- Make sure that at least 1.5 litres of the water you drink is still.

- Make sure the water is slightly chilled or, ideally, at room temperature.

- Make sure the water is fresh – a bottle newly opened that day, a glassful freshly poured from the filter jug or the tap.

- Make sure your water intake is spread out over the whole day – say, 1 large glassful each hour.

- Make sure you replace any water lost – every time you drink a cup of coffee, have at least the same amount in water. This will be in addition to your 2 litres. Do the same when drinking alcohol: match every glass with a glass of water.

- If you exercise, make sure you drink throughout the workout and after, but don't count this as part of your 2-litre intake per day – exercise requires much more fluid.

- Replace tea or coffee with hot water – it means you still go through the same ritual of heating the kettle, and so on, but without the diuretic effect of the caffeine.

- Herbal tea, still water, fizzy water, and water mixed with fruit juice all count as water. Coffee, tea, alcohol, and fruit cordials do not count as water.

- Keep your water fresh. Don't leave a bottle of water in your car in the summer and drink from it over a period of several weeks. You need to make sure that it doesn't end up teeming with bacteria from being left in a hot, damp environment.

- Tap, bottled, reversed osmosis, oxygenated, filtered – any water counts as long as it is pure water.

NB: If you drink too much too soon, you literally 'drown' your body. You cannot use a lot of water all at the same time: you will overload your system and actually end up flushing out essential nutrients and foods. That can be damaging. If you are exercising, you should still drink, but not in such large amounts that you are flushing through essential sugars needed for exercise. This will make you feel a little faint.

WHEN TO DRINK WATER

There is a technique that will ensure you do drink your full water quota without spending your life in the toilet, lying in bed half the night thinking about going to the toilet, staying late at the office until you have downed the remaining 1 litre you forgot to drink during the day, and so on.

- As soon as you get up, drink a glassful of water. This will hydrate you from the night before.

- For breakfast, always drink a mug of hot water and fresh lemon juice to cleanse your system – this counts towards your water requirement.

- Every time you go to the toilet, take 8 mouthfuls of water to replace the fluids lost.

- Every time someone offers to make you a cup of tea or coffee, just ask for a cup of hot water or herbal tea.

- Before lunch make sure you drink a glassful of water. This will dampen your appetite and stop you drinking with your food, which decreases absorption of nutrients.

- Before supper, drink another glass of water for the same reason.

- Make sure you have had at least 1.5 litres of water before 6 p.m.

- Visit the toilet before you get into bed, but have your last small glassful before going to sleep – just 4 or 5 mouthfuls.

- Enjoy your deep and restful sleep.

It may seem silly to be told how to drink water. But if you simply go from drinking nothing to drinking 2 litres in a short space of time, it will be uncomfortable for your digestion. And it could actually be quite dangerous if you 'flood' your body, which will prevent it from absorbing the essential nutrients that it needs.

A TASTE FOR WATER

If you have only been drinking tap water and haven't given it a second thought, then just carry on as you are. The last thing the Water Detox programme should do is to reduce your current levels of water intake.

The aim of the programme is either to get you to start drinking water in the first place or to get you to increase the amounts you currently drink. If you do drink a good amount of water per day, then congratulations – you are already well on the way to total Water Detox. I hope you are already aware of the benefits. In any case, this programme will point out a few ways that you may not have considered of getting more water into your life and how water can actually affect you.

Just as there are many different varieties of soft drink, alcoholic drink and hot drink, there are many varieties of 'water drink'. That may sound odd. How could water be as varied as, say, wine? With this, of course, there are different grape varieties from different regions within the country of origin. And look at coffee: there must be hundreds of different beans to taste, from Blue Mountain, Kenyan, Colombian caffeinated, to decaffeinated and so on. You can ring the changes with tea, too – herbal, green, black, Oolong, Earl Grey, Assam, Darjeeling ... the list goes on, and you can probably recite all these from the top of your head.

But water seems to be different. If we talk about water, the immediate thought is that it's simply water. We don't give water a chance to be appealing. Yet if you just scratch the surface of the water industry, you will immediately see that the choices available to us are just as varied and amazing as they are within all the other industries we have looked at and mentioned above.

So, to say you don't like water and that you find it boring or without taste is to say that you have no real knowledge of how varied and different the water market is. Not only are there hundreds of different types, there are hundreds of different origins, sources, flavours – yes, flavours – and even textures on the palate, known as 'mouth feel'. So read on. You may just stumble upon a water that was designed with you in mind, your need for purification and your budget.

Which Water?

There are hundreds of stories telling us how dangerous it is to drink tap water. There are also hundreds of stories telling us that we are totally wasting our money on buying bottled water. We are informed that tap water is full of pesticides and pollution and we are then told that bottled water, unless extremely fresh, will be full of toxins transferred from the plastic bottle if not kept in laboratory conditions.

So what, really and truly, is the difference, and which is the best for us?

In my view, water is the most important aspect of this argument. As long as you are drinking it, you are all right. It is better to be drinking water, whatever the source, than not drinking it at all. So – as I've said – if tap water is your tipple, there is no problem. If you don't drink water because you have heard that tap water is bad and you are not prepared to pay for bottled then start drinking tap water now. The benefits of hydration far outweigh any risks indicated by a few rumours and stories. Having said this, please read the 'Tap Water' section below carefully to see what it can contain, as you may choose to filter it. This is up to you: I'm aiming for a balanced view of the options.

What about all the different kinds of water?

Water comes in more types than just tap, still or fizzy. There are many definitions, and thanks to regulations, they do actually help:

- Drinking water

- Mineral water

- Natural mineral water

- Purified water

- Distilled water

- Sparkling water

- Spring water

- Natural spring water

Once you are drinking water on a regular basis, you can become more discerning and go for price, taste and content. Just as with any drink, there will be some waters you like and some you don't. If this hasn't been a consideration for you, then you can do some home tests and you might just discover a taste you like so much that drinking your 2 litres a day will be a breeze. Equally, if you have never drunk your full quota because you don't like the taste, don't give up. Do some investigations and find one that you really enjoy.

HINTS AND TIPS TO FIND YOUR TIPPLE

Tap Water

Tap water is our lifeline. We use it for washing, bathing, cooking and drinking. Some areas have what we call hard water and some soft water. If you travel to a different part of the country, tap water will have a different taste and smell, and if you travel around the world you'll hear the constant refrain 'don't drink the water'. So it's variable stuff, both locally and globally.

It is possible to find out what is in your tap water by approaching the local water authority. It can give you a water analysis for your area. This may mean a lot to you, or nothing whatsoever, but if it means that you drink more water then please do it! It is normal for domestic water supplies to contain trace metals, fluorides, herbicides and pesticides. It is also common folklore that the water we drink has already been through 70 other people before it gets to our glass.

Tap water has undergone strict examination and must fulfil exacting safety standards before it can be supplied to the public. So in Britain and most of the West, the tap water we have is safe. If you wish you can make it even safer. Filtration of domestic water will remove even the trace elements that remain in the general supply. If you feel this is necessary, try the various methods available. Do remember that anything in the supply is in trace amounts and cleared as safe for consumption. Indeed, the government has even mooted a plan to put essential vitamin nutrients into our tap water to make sure that we are all getting them. It could be even better for us than we imagined ...

Meanwhile let's look at what the stuff from our tap actually contains.

Aluminium

This is crucial to our bodies as it helps to protect the immune system. Aluminium is commonly used in the purification and treatment of water. It gets into our water supply through acid rain and through rainwater running over soil and rocks with high aluminium content and into the water table. It can be found in older water storage equipment. Excess consumption or absorption of aluminium has been reported to contribute to the incidence of Alzheimer's disease, but only in very high amounts.

Bacteria and germs

Britain's domestic water supplies are sophisticated and safe enough to be able to guarantee that waterborne diseases are virtually non-existent, if we drink fresh water directly from the tap and don't leave it in a container or vessel before consumption. There have been very rare cases of people becoming ill from tap water bacteria content. There can be incidents where something gets into the water and contaminates it, but the water authorities are very quick to cease supply and take emergency measures until it is safe to drink from the tap again. Our bodies are used to the make-up of our local water. Drinking water in some other countries may not always be quite so safe, or may have such a different chemical make-up that, although it is not dangerous, it can cause a temporary upset stomach.

Chlorine

We use chlorine to ensure that all bacteria are cleansed and eliminated from our domestic drinking water. You can often smell slight traces of chlorine when you run the tap. Chlorine is safe and we are probably more familiar with its use in public swimming pools to kill germs and neutralise water. The only problem might lie in drinking large amounts of chlorinated water, as high levels of chlorine may just kill off the good bacteria in our intestines – the intestinal flora and fauna that protect our guts.

Fluoride

If you have ever been to the dentist or are familiar with the contents of toothpaste, you will have heard of fluoride – in its more common usage. Many local authorities add fluoride to drinking water for that very purpose, to develop young teeth and gums and bones. However, in some European countries the addition of fluoride to the local water supply is actually illegal. It is supposed to prevent tooth decay, but it is also supposed to cause heart problems and birth defects. Clearly not enough is known about this substance for the argument to be weighted one way or the other. The trace amounts in domestic water sources should be OK, but you might wish to check to see if your local supply has added amounts.

Hard and soft water

Some areas of the country are reported to have hard water and some soft. I come from Manchester and as a child remember going to visit relatives in Essex and finding the taste of the water totally unbearable. The water I was familiar with was 'soft' water, but the water in Essex was 'hard'.

The differences between the two are quite simple but also quite substantial. Hard water contains higher levels of calcium and magnesium, and soft water has higher levels of sodium. Hard water is better for the heart, so even though soft water seems more palatable to some people it isn't always the most beneficial. You can soften the water you bathe in, but leave the water you drink as hard as you can.

Lead

Lead in the water is not good. Lead is poisonous and the body cannot process or eliminate it. The lead builds up and can eventually lead to ill health. Water from domestic sources has a relatively low lead content, but by the time water reaches our taps the amount of lead in it can be higher – especially if you live in London or very old cities and towns, where the local plumbing network and system will probably be made of lead piping. Our old-fashioned domestic water supply means that the water arrives with more lead than when it left the purification plant. You should always run the tap before pouring yourself a drink of water, as the water that has been standing in the pipes all night may well have absorbed more metals than are good for us.

Nitrates

Nitrates are substances found in sewage and some chemical fertilisers. They can enter the water supply via these sources. Whatever the source, they are not good for us in any way. Nitrates are considered by some to cause some cancers, and in high doses can lead to so-called 'blue baby syndrome' in infants.

Pesticides, herbicides and drugs

No matter how sophisticated our water purification plants, they seem to be unable totally to cleanse the water of trace elements of a number of prescription drugs and drugs that replace or regulate hormones. Pesticides and herbicides are also left in the water in minimal amounts.

These facts are not meant to be a scare tactic, but it is worth considering the content of your tap water if you intend to drink only from your domestic supply. If you are looking to drink tap water as a fallback option, then I wouldn't even think about it. But if it is to be your only source, you may want to know exactly where you stand.

Obviously, detoxification is about cleansing your body and eliminating any waste or damaging products. As you've now seen, drinking tap water during detoxification is not the purest approach but if it is the only way I can encourage you to drink water, then I can only recommend it. But all is not lost: you can actually clean your own water, ready for drinking and sparkling clean – well nearly.

Cleansing Tap Water

Before deciding that your only option is to go out and buy bottled water in whatever form you can – and we will discuss this soon – you may want to look at ways to cleanse the 'free' and convenient water you receive via your tap.

Filtered water

There are many ways to filter tap water: filters you buy from the supermarket right through to filters you have installed into your domestic supply so that what actually comes out of your tap is totally filtered already. Here are some of the differences:

Carbon filters The filters available to drop into water jugs at home are usually carbon granules in a tube, and are relatively cheap. The water is poured through the filter to cleanse it of chlorine, and improve the smell and taste. It neutralises the water rather than deep-cleanses it. Carbon-filtered water does not lose the normal nutrients and minerals found in tap water as they are too small to be eliminated. Filtering water in this way is quite easy but fairly labour intensive. Many of the jugs or systems have a shelf life for the filter that should be carefully and strictly observed: discard it as soon as it reaches its expiry date. If you don't do this, you are likely to be filtering your fresh tap water through carbon grains full of absorbed chemicals and chlorine and, potentially, bacteria or moulds – yuck.

Do check the filter system before you buy. Some will just remove stale tastes and smell, while others claim to eliminate low-impact contamination.

Installed water filters A lot easier to use and keep updated than the jug filters, but not the most effective system available. These systems perform the very same function as the charcoal filter jugs except they are plumbed in next to your cold water supply so you no longer need to fill a jug in order to clean your water – you simply turn on your new tap. You only need to change the filter once or twice a year depending on usage. Less effort but initially more expensive.

Reverse osmosis This system is also one that you have plumbed in to your water supply and you usually end up with an extra tap or spout next to your cold water tap. You will also need room in your kitchen cupboards for a water tank for reverse osmosis purification. Reverse osmosis systems claim to be able to thoroughly clean the drinking water. Water is processed through a semipermeable membrane that collects all chemicals, all bacteria, pesticides and herbicides, any viruses and any metal content. The downside is that it cleanses the water of all the beneficial nutrients as well, so your water is squeaky clean! This system is expensive but extremely effective. If you have any concerns about your water supply or your health then this system will almost certainly guarantee totally clean water.

So much for improving tap water. What about if you decide to go out and buy the stuff?

Bottled Waters

Some bottled waters may not be any cleaner than filtered tap waters. There are many different categories and stipulations attached to bottling water as a product, and they are not always as clear as they seem.

There are no rules or regulations as to the metal, mineral or salt content of bottled waters. The difference in content is extreme. If you buy bottled waters, you will be aware of the differing tastes, and will have your favourites and also some that you cannot stomach. This is all to do with the waters' varying contents.

Table water, bottled drinking water, mineral water, spring water, distilled water – all these are names for differing levels of purity in the water. Some are quite simply tap water in a bottle and some are rigorously tested and monitored for purity and cleanliness – but which is which?

Flavoured waters

Bottled, flavoured waters are not permitted on the Water Detox. They will almost certainly be full of sugar, artificial flavourings and sweeteners. The only flavoured water allowed is water you flavour yourself with natural juices, herbs, or vegetables.

To fizz or not to fizz

Nearly all the categories of water we describe below come in still and fizzy varieties. The fizzy varieties then split into two further categories – naturally sparkling and carbonated.

If you really wish to drink fizzy water, the naturally sparkling variety (naturally carbonated) is best, although in many cases the natural sparkle is lost and needs to be replaced before it is served to us from the bottle. Try to keep to only 2 or 3 glasses of fizz a day. Not only is the naturalness of the 'sparkling' questionable, but it is likely to cause bloating.

The other kind of fizzy water is still water that has had carbon pumped into it, and this is not desirable. It can actually prevent our bodies from absorbing all the minerals and nutrients in the water itself. It will also cause bloating, and there are some reports that it can even cause cellulite!

So on the whole, it's best to stick to still, flat, *sin gas or eau naturelle* when you're buying bottled.

Table water, spring water and drinking water

These kinds of water are of the same standard as tap water. The water is usually bottled in a safe, sterilised container for consumption. The water can be sourced from natural spring outlets or mains outlets. It can be filtered, it can be treated and it can have been blended with a number of types of water. You just pay for someone to bottle it and hopefully treat it in one or another of those ways.

Purified water

Purified water is any water that has been distilled or filtered via reverse osmosis (see page 30–31). Virtually all the nutrients have been taken out of this water, so it is not very beneficial to drink. Purified water or distilled waters are designed for use in kettles or electrical implements to prevent the build-up of scale on the inside. All bottled waters should be stored carefully and consumed well within their 'best before' date. Waters stored in plastic bottles in the sunlight may develop a tainted flavour, and if the bottle has been opened or even if a drink has been taken from the bottle, the potential for bacteria to develop in it is high. It should be drunk or used when it is still as fresh as possible.

Natural mineral water

Natural mineral water must come from an underground source. Nothing can be added or taken out, but the bacteria in it must be eliminated. It has no minimum mineral content stipulations attached to it, but it must maintain its contents. It can be carbonated. In some countries natural mineral water is the same as spring water. Italian and French spring waters undergo the same stipulations that mineral waters in Britain do. The term 'mineral' is used because the water has travelled through many underground routes to get to the bottle. It has travelled over, under and through many different rock formations, and each of these types of rock contributes to the mineral content of the water. It is this 'route' that is generally used to try to persuade us of the purity/taste/mineral content, and make us buy it! I'm sure you've heard or read the ads:

'Flowing from a source in the heart of this beautiful region of France'
'Originating from a beautiful wooded valley'
'Natural rainwater from Australia'
'Fresh from the Canadian Rockies' – and so on.

Whatever the source, the minerals in mineral water are actually very valuable in our diet and for our general health. If you choose a mineral water on your Water Detox that can supplement any essential minerals from your foods, this can only be an advantage.

The most common minerals are shown below, with their health benefits.

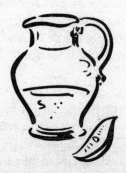

Mineral	Benefits
Calcium	Calcium is essential for growth and strength of bones and teeth. It also helps the brain communicate with the body and the muscles. We can get as much calcium from our daily mineral water as we do from milk, and it's totally detox!
Magnesium	Magnesium helps with strong bones and teeth. It also promotes good heart health and great circulation. It is used in the body for most cell activity and is also essential for the proper function of calcium.
Sodium	We know that sodium helps to balance the levels of fluid inside the body. The main problem is that we have too much of it so low amounts are preferable in your mineral water of choice.
Potassium	Potassium works with sodium in regulating the body's water content. It helps expel excess sodium, which in turn helps prevent high blood pressure.
Chloride	This works with both potassium and sodium to regulate water levels in the body.
Bicarbonates	Help to regulate the pH balance of the body.
Sulphates	Said to promote good hormone balance, and aid in assimilation of vitamins and proteins. Foods high in sulphur have also shown an ability to decrease the risk of cancers and blood clots.

From this description, you can see that it is probably safe to summarise that the only water worth paying for on health grounds is natural mineral water. It is guaranteed to have a mineral content, in every bottle. You should choose your mineral water according to your own particular taste. Some waters are far too salty for my taste, while others taste really refreshing. Buy a few different ones over a period of time and discover the many flavours of water.

You may also wish to consider the recommendations of the Bluebird Restaurant in London. Their sommelier recommends a salty water to drink with marine fish, to give seawater overtones, and a slightly sweeter water to go with meat, to lend earthy overtones. Whatever your taste and whatever your dish, make sure that water is a main consideration.

There is, of course, also a huge range of bottles available. Have some fun and choose your fresh mineral water according to the bottle, blue, green, tall or short. Adorn your table with an exotic bottle and see how much more quickly your guests will guzzle. Once the water is finished, use the bottle to place a candle in and have an instant table decoration for your next gathering – your own personalised water bar. *Très chic*.

A matter of convenience

Bottled water has another prime advantage. It is often much easier to carry a bottle of water with you to ensure that you are keeping your water levels up than to expect to be able to get to a tap and find a glass if you are not at home. Carrying water means that as soon as you feel thirsty or would like a drink you can do it then and there. Having a lid on a bottle of water ensures that it stays clean if you leave it by your bed or on your desk. It also means that your computer keyboard, magazine and bedroom carpet don't get an inconvenient watering that needs mopping up when you knock your glass over.

Using bottled water is also a good way to check how much you are drinking each day. To try to drink 2 litres per day is a good goal, but to know how many glasses of water that means is another thing entirely. When you drink glasses of water at someone else's house or try to add up the water content of everything else you have consumed, you are likely to fail to drink the whole 2 litres.

But if you take 2 litre bottles of water out of the fridge each morning and drink them throughout the day, you will be left in no doubt as to how much you have consumed. I am not suggesting that you need to carry the full 2 litres about with you first thing in the morning, but you could have one for the morning and one for the afternoon. Most large bottles are 1.5 litres and these are quite heavy. As an alternative you could just buy a 500-millilitre bottle each morning and then fill it up 3 more times from the tap throughout the day. You could buy your 1.5-litre bottle in the morning near to work and then have your final 500 millilitres at home in the evening. Whatever you do, you can see that it's actually pretty easy to get your full 2-litre quota each day.

HOW OUR BODIES USE WATER

Water, as we know, is a cleanser. But how, exactly, does our body use this water, and what does it need it for?

The Liver

The liver is our largest internal organ. Its main functions are regulating metabolism and detoxification or cleansing. The liver takes in the waste substances or 'poisons' that enter our bodies when we consume foods and liquids, or absorb from the environment and by inhalation. The liver converts them for us to use, eliminate or store. It controls levels of fats and glucose in the blood. It fights against infection, cleaning bacteria from the blood and body. It processes and stores all our necessary vitamins and iron and helps repair damaged tissues.

So the liver is incredibly busy, working on our behalf to cleanse the body. It acts as damage limitation, so anything we cannot use or that arrives in a dangerous or damaging state is processed, disarmed or neutralised and then, if possible, used to its best advantage. Any products for elimination are then made water soluble and passed out into the intestines for final elimination.

There are, of course, many things we eat and breathe that the body simply must eliminate as soon as possible, and the liver takes full responsibility for this. These substances include alcohol, additives, caffeine, smoke, fizzy drinks, exhaust fumes, drugs (prescribed and non-prescribed) and anything that we really don't need but that has become an integral part of our lives.

If we constantly feed our bodies these 'useless' products, the liver has a hard job to keep up with processing them. It is incredibly adept at flushing them through but just like our own lives, if we constantly add to our 'to do' list without ever stopping, the workload becomes unmanageable. If the liver has to work too hard over too long a period of time, it will become tired and sluggish. It will take longer to process the wastes and then, unless we give it a rest in the form of a detox programme, we can start to develop minor illnesses that can eventually become major. These can range from tiredness and lethargy, to jaundice, exhaustion or even alcohol poisoning and liver failure.

It should therefore come as no surprise that cutting down useless foods and drinks, or even eliminating them, and adding water and nutritious foods, can only serve to develop super-efficient and rested livers.

The Kidneys

The kidneys are the body's other cleansing stars. They take care of all matters fluid within the body, cleansing the blood and keeping the fluid balanced by regulating potassium and sodium levels. They also perform the important function of regulating pH – the balance of acidity and alkalinity within the body. Any of these areas in imbalance can cause huge problems.

After cleansing the blood, the kidneys pass the waste materials into the urinary system for elimination. If the kidneys are overworked, we can get kidney infections, kidney stones and bladder stones. Obviously these are very serious conditions, but on a day-to-day basis we will just feel tired as the body attempts to concentrate on the normal processing of wastes.

The Lymph System

The lymph system is the body's waste disposal system. Everything we consume is processed by certain organs, as we can see, but the lymph system is on patrol throughout the body picking up infections, germs, waste or toxic substances and making sure that they are eliminated and not allowed back into the blood system or circulation.

Lymph absorbs dead cells, excess fluids and other waste products and takes them to the lymph nodes. Here the waste is filtered and is eventually fed to the eliminatory organs – skin, liver, or kidneys – to be passed out via perspiration, faeces or urine.

The Skin

The skin is the body's largest external organ. It is one of the first ports of call for toxins, sweating out waste products such as water, salts, uric acid, ammonia and urea. The skin is like a huge colander; all the waste comes out and the goodness remains behind. If we are overloading our body's internal cleansing systems or even just overdoing it a bit, then the skin is one of the first organs to show the telltale signs. We get pale or slightly yellow or grey, we get spots and we lose any form of rosy glow.

The skin also helps to regulate body temperature through its ability to sweat. If we get hot our bodies produce sweat to cool down. If we get cold our blood vessels dilate and reduce the blood flow at the surface of the skin down into the internal organs. This prevents heat loss. If we are dehydrated we often feel cold, as the body cannot perform its function well, and if we are too hot and dehydrated then the body cannot cool as efficiently, as it has no water stocks to use.

The skin mirrors what is going on internally, so if you hear 'You look great', 'You are glowing', or 'You look pale' or 'You don't look good', you can be pretty sure of your state of inner health. The face can tell a thousand things and the most important of these is how well you are. The Chinese will even use the face and skin to help diagnose ailments. Chinese face reading looks at lines and coloration, and there are certain areas that are said to directly reflect the activity of the digestive system and liver – notably, the chin. So, if you have a spotty chin, let your detox begin!

The Lungs

Not normally associated with cleansing, the lungs filter the very air we breathe, which is why we can get through living in the city with all the fumes and toxins attacking us. The lungs will disarm any harmful products in the air and help the body process and eliminate them.

Our lungs are full of little air sacs – you imagine them as little vacuum bags. They fill with the air we breathe and they exchange oxygen and carbon dioxide. We breathe in oxygen and the lungs expel the waste water and carbon dioxide. Along with air, we tend to breathe in a whole host of useless and poisonous substances as well: car fumes, cigarette smoke, pesticides, chemicals from household products and perfumes, and so on. The air we breathe is much more than fresh air.

Cigarette smoke is one of the toxins most commonly associated with the lungs. The tar from cigarettes cannot be expelled and so builds up inside the lungs. The build-up can eventually cause congestion and lung failure.

The Intestines

The liver and lymph need to pass waste somewhere within the body for elimination. Skin can expel toxins directly, and the lungs can expel gases directly, while the kidneys pass fluids and waste to the urinary system via the bladder. But all other solid waste needs to go via the intestines. As well as picking up waste from the organs of elimination, the intestines also directly eliminate solids from the process of digestion. The food we eat passes through the stomach and into the intestines: all the goodness is absorbed into the bloodstream and then waste is pushed through and out the other end.

In a normal, healthy body, the digestive process, from consumption to elimination, should be approximately 8 hours. In bodies that are undernourished and dehydrated, following an unhealthy diet, or even just stressed and overworked, the process will take over 24 hours. As the body's processing slows down, we find that the intestines become 'backed up'. Constipation and excess gas are just some of the unpleasant and unhealthy side effects.

How Does Water Cleanse?

Every one of the functions described above can be improved, made more efficient or speeded up if we add water to the body. Each and every organ and system – liver, kidneys, lungs, skin and intestines – uses water as its vehicle for cleansing in some way or another. If you don't drink enough water the process slows down: urine becomes dark and pungent, you become constipated, with hard stools, you get infections and swollen glands, and your skin goes pale and grey. If you add water, and then start to supply your body on a regular basis with the amount it actually needs to function efficiently, everything changes: clear pH-balanced urine, efficient bowel movement and cleansed intestines, a healthy immune system ready to fight any infection, and glowing, radiant skin.

You can start to see that we really should consider dehydration as a very serious illness that we can cure by simply drinking more water each day.

Look at the symptoms in the box on the next page. Do any of these seem familiar to you? Do any of them ring true and you haven't been able to fathom why all this time? Well, now you know. It is incredibly common to have one or more of these symptoms on a fairly continuous basis and to have accepted them so much that they are now your 'norm'. Drinking water means you can wave goodbye to them. Remember, we are 75 per cent water, the brain is around 80 per cent, muscles 75 per cent, plasma 91 per cent, blood 92 per cent, bones 22 per cent, and cells up to 70 per cent. No wonder we feel ill when we fail to drink enough!

Some simple side effects of dehydration

Lack of concentration	Colds	Bladder infections
Tiredness	Water retention	Pale skin
Higher stress levels	Cellulite	Spots/congestion
Anxiety	Bloating	Confusion
Depression	Nausea	Headaches
Dry skin	Indigestion	Aching joints
Itchy skin	Pungent urine	
Illnesses	Painful urination	

2

The 18-Day H₂0 Nutrition Programme

W E CONSUME A LOT OF TOXINS when we eat and drink. There is also contamination from pollutants, germs and fumes, but the main culprits are foods. Our eating habits have become incredibly varied and adventurous and the food manufacturers have done their best to make sure we can get hold of whatever we want to eat whenever we want. This has led to the use of preservatives, colourings and additives. Our bodies cannot use them and so they are also considered toxins.

HOW WATER FEEDS US

The body works hard to process these toxins through the liver, kidneys, lymph and the rest of the cleansing system, so it can excrete them. If the build-up of toxins outweighs the body's ability to process them, the body slows down to cope with the workload. If we detox, then we give our body a rest, so it can eventually clear all the waste and start with a clean slate. We feel fabulous and rejuvenated. The body has been given the chance to get back in control instead of trying to catch up all the time.

Water is an essential part of this cleansing process. We've seen how vital it is to drink enough water to benefit. Eating the right foods is very important too. Many of our foods contain over 50 per cent water, some as much as 95 per cent. Following a programme that concentrates on these foods will inevitably lead to optimum hydration and therefore optimum detoxification.

However, it is important to know that just because we eat foods containing a high percentage of water, it doesn't mean that we no longer need to drink water or fluids throughout the day. The normal levels recommended for drinking are always the 'minimum' levels, as this reflects the fact that we are expected to gain some fluids through our daily eating programmes. Following the Water Detox programme will simply mean that we guarantee the right levels of water, or exceed them.

It should come as no surprise that foods we commonly associate with detoxification and cleansing are also the foods that are high in water content – the two go hand in hand. The main difference between the two is that in traditional detox programmes we eat a certain amount of diuretic foods, which cause us to urinate more frequently and copiously. This process is necessary for the cleansing process to work well. In the Water Detox programme we will be eating foods that are so high in water that we have no need for diuretics – the fluid levels alone will take care of that quite nicely. We do need to make sure our kidneys are looked after, as they will be working overtime to keep the fluid levels and the potassium/sodium levels regulated and healthy.

The following common foods have at least 50 per cent water content. They are listed in tables to encourage you to make sure you get the right balance of foods during your Water Detox. Combining detoxification with total hydration kills two birds with one stone. It speeds up the process and aids the body's route to recovery. It is no surprise that the Water Detox is effective in 18 days and not the usual 30.

Following the programme for just 18 days means that you should reach optimum hydration in a very short time. The thing to remember is that you cannot eat anything that is not in the programme, as it may well slow up the process or even reverse it!

I haven't included diuretics in the Water Detox for a very particular reason: we are trying to get water in, not encourage it to go out. The body is extremely efficient in getting rid of used water but we don't want to add anything that means we banish water from the system before our bodies have had the chance to put it to full use. Diuretics in any form are not appropriate for the programme. The common rule of thumb with these products is that for every amount of diuretic you take you will lose the same amount of water or more – never less. So if you drink a cup of coffee (which acts as a diuretic) every hour, you will lose over a cup of water every hour.

The most common culprits are unfortunately the most commonly consumed foods and drinks in our diet. Certain activities can have a diuretic effect too. They should be eliminated or managed for the next 18 days.

WATER-LOSS CULPRITS

Coffee/Caffeine/Colas/Stimulant Drinks

Often people say they don't drink coffee or tea, but then they let slip that they have a few cans of cola each day. Or they argue that tea contains less caffeine than coffee. Whatever the argument, it isn't worth it.

Any drink containing caffeine will not only help to dehydrate you, but it will also leave a residue for your body to clean up. On top of this it will give you a temporary caffeine/sugar high that will result in a slump in energy pretty soon afterwards. You must not have these during the programme. They are full of toxins and they act as diuretics.

Alcohol

Just as with caffeine, every glass of alcohol you drink means you lose a glass of water from your body. The alcohol in drinks positively encourages your body to move water out. This explains the queue for the toilets in most clubs, bars and pubs. If you can match your glass of alcohol with a glass of water then you will be keeping the balance, but you will still need to make sure that the required 2 litres is still on the agenda. Alcohol is not part of the 18-Day H_2O Nutrition Programme.

Activity/Exercise

We know that exercise makes us sweat, but that is just the physical external way of knowing that we are losing fluids. The increase in muscle use, rate of metabolism and circulation requires more fluids to work efficiently. This internal work doesn't stop the moment we stop exercising. If you are working hard physically, or working out, your body will be getting rid of precious water levels. You must make sure that you add an extra litre of water per hour of exercise. Drink the water throughout the period of exertion and not just at the end or start. You must allow your body time to produce essential salts before drowning it in water. Again, a glassful an hour is a good measure for normal day-to-day activity, so a glassful or 10 mouthfuls per 5 minutes is a good measure for exertion or exercise.

Exercise and activity is very good for us and extremely good for detoxification. It speeds up the cleansing process. Don't cut out activity – just increase your water consumption.

Sleeping

Don't forget that when we sleep, we lose water through sweating and normal metabolism. But obviously, as we are sleeping, we are not replacing these fluids. Indeed, having a lot to drink just before going to bed will have you up in the night to go to the toilet. If you are anything like me, you will find yourself lying awake trying to convince yourself that you don't need to go and that the feeling will go away.

Make sure that when you get up in the morning you have a good-sized glass of water to rehydrate. Start a new bottle, pour it fresh from the filter, or let the tap run so that it is sparkling and cool – don't be tempted to drink from the stale water by your bed. That is no longer fresh and invigorated and needs to be disposed of in a plant pot or in the garden – don't waste it, just don't bother to drink it.

Make sure your breakfast is high in water content. Yoghurt and fruits are great for this. Make the first meal of the day 'high hydration'.

Illness or Recovery

The body works hard to heal itself, and the immune system goes into overdrive if we have an infection or a virus. We get a temperature and we feel lethargic and tired. This is the body's way of telling us to rest so that it can concentrate on getting better. When we have a temperature, we become dehydrated quicker, so we need to keep fluid levels ideal to allow the body to work in optimum conditions. Obviously, we hope you will not be ill during the programme but if you do get a bug, then remember to hydrate to recover and recuperate.

Stimulant Foods – Curries, Spices, Juniper, Dandelion and Nettle Teas

There are many herbs that encourage us to expel fluids and many foods that increase the heat in our bodies and therefore use up more fluids than normal. Make sure that if you are eating any of these or are taking any remedies that contain diuretic products that you increase your own fluid intake. These foods are delicious and nutritious but you may want to exclude them for the next 18 days to give yourself the best chance of full hydration.

Urination

This is certainly the most obvious form of fluid loss! When we go to the toilet we should always remember to replace what we have just got rid of. A good rule is to drink 8 mouthfuls of water for every emptied bladder. This will immediately replenish stocks and keep you working at full hydration.

Once we have established what foods will hydrate and which will dehydrate, we can go on to devise our eating plan.

How to eat (and drink)

Foods

You can have: oily fish, oils, yoghurts, potatoes, beans and pulses, vegetables, fruits, rice and salads.

This list of foods you can have seems quite restrictive if we just mention them generally, but don't worry: the list expands hugely if you actually look at what they include:

Fish	Oils	Cheeses & Yoghurts	Potatoes
Mackerel	Olive	Roquefort	Jacket potatoes
Herring	Sunflower	Chevre	Sweet potatoes
Sardines	Sesame	Ricotta	New potatoes
Anchovies	Walnut	Feta	Yams
Whitebait	Grapeseed	Pecorino Romano	Jerusalem artichokes
Salmon	Nut	Manchego	
Tuna		All goat's and sheep's cheeses and yoghurts	

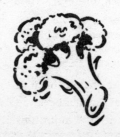

Pulses

Aduki
Black beans
Flageolet
Kidney
Cannellini
Pinto
Mung
Chickpeas
Haricot
Puy lentils
Red lentils
Green lentils
Split peas

Cabbages & Greens

Spring greens
Cabbage –
    Savoy cabbage
    Red cabbage
    White cabbage
Brussels sprouts
Cauliflower
Broccoli –
    Green
    Long stem
    Purple sprouting

Onions

Spanish onions
White onions
Red onions
Leeks
Shallots
Spring onions
Garlic
Chives

Tomatoes

Cherry
Plum
Beef
Normal

Rice

Brown
Short grain
    brown
Red Camargue
Wild

Fruits

Grapes
Grapefruit
Pineapples
Oranges
Lemons
Limes
Peaches
Apricots
Apples
Pears
Kiwi fruit
Mangoes
Passionfruit
Cherries
Raspberries
Strawberries
Blackberries
Blackcurrants
Redcurrants
Blueberries
Cranberries
Plums

Salad Vegetables

Lettuce –
    Iceberg
    Webb
    Endive
    Cos
Rocket
Pak choy
Chinese leaf
Radicchio
Lollo rosso
Lambs lettuce
Watercress
Spinach
Cress
Fennel
Avocados
Radish
Celery
Peppers
Cucumbers

Other Vegetables

Beetroot
Courgettes
Turnips
Parsnips
Swedes
Pumpkins
Squashes
Beans –
    Haricot
    Broad
    Runner
Peas –
    Mangetout
    Sugar snap
    Fresh
    Frozen
Sweetcorn
Baby sweetcorn
Okra/ladies' fingers
Carrots
Asparagus

Teas	Herbs	Seasoning	Nuts
Herbal –	Coriander	Fresh ground pepper	Any nuts of choice
Peppermint	Chervil		but in moderation
Jasmine	Chicory		
Ginseng	Dill		
Chamomile	Fennel		
Nettle	Marjoram		
Fennel	Oregano		
Ginger	Parsley		
Green	Tarragon		
Raspberry leaf	Thyme		
And many more			

The cheeses and oils do not always have a 50 per cent water content, but I've included them to ensure that you are getting a balanced diet. The sheep's and goat's products are much more digestible by the human body and much more tolerable than dairy products to many people. For this reason we are using 'non-dairy' in the H_2O Nutrition Programme.

For each of the 18 days you must:

- Drink at least 2 litres of water in pure, plain form.

- Eat at least 3 full meals a day or 5 small meals a day.

- Eat at least 5 portions of fruits each day.

- Eat at least 5 portions of vegetables per day.

- Eat at least 2 portions of fish, beans or pulses per day.

- Eat at least 1 portion of rice per day.

- Eat at least 1 portion of oil or cheese per day.

All foods are freely available to eat throughout the programme but the above is the absolute minimum. You must make sure you are eating a balanced diet, and not too much fat and oil or too few vegetables and fruits.

Cooking Methods

If you want to keep your foods moist, succulent and with the right level of hydration you must use the right cooking methods. Whichever one you choose, you should always aim to use any of the juices, essences or fluids that come out of the foods for dressings or sauces or as gravy to pour back over them.

Eating raw foods will maintain total fluid levels and total nutrients. You should aim to eat half of your foods each day raw. These can be fruits or vegetables, but obviously not rice or potatoes!

Rice is excellent, though, as it arrives dried and then we add water to it for cooking – ideal for hydration.

Parcel steaming and ordinary steaming are both methods that will leave your food juicy and hydrated. Indeed, they add water to it. Stir frying, grilling, griddling and baking will preserve water levels too, especially if, as I've already suggested, you use any fluids that are thrown off in cooking in gravies, or poured back over the foods before you eat them. They are healthy methods as you don't need to add excess fats – stir frying only requires minuscule amounts of oil, so don't overdo it unless you are using this as your fat intake for the day.

The absolute best way to ensure that you don't lose fluids during cooking is to make sure that you add them! Making soups, stews, smoothies and long drinks is definitely something to aim for. Not only does this increase the fluid content, but also it ensures that you don't lose any nutrients.

Fluids

Any fluid you drink on top of your daily 2 litres is just exactly that – an addition. Do not think that having a mug of herbal tea is 'instead of'. It is really a bonus, and remember, the *minimum* water intake is 2 litres a day, so anything extra is extremely beneficial and nutritious.

RECIPE SUGGESTIONS

The following recipes are just a few suggestions as to how you can make your Water Detox as tasty as it is nutritious. If you want to experiment in the kitchen then there should be something on the next few pages to get your creative juices flowing. The recipes are in quantities for one person for a small meal. If you are having 3 meals a day rather than 5, then you can increase the amounts to suit. If you don't want to follow the recipes, then simply take the food list to the supermarket, buy the foods and come home to experiment and surprise yourself. If you have friends for dinner they will only suspect that you are an incredibly healthy and creative host/hostess. Try something you may never have tried before and see how wonderful it feels to be on the H_2O Nutrition Programme.

If you have no interest in cooking, remember that you can still enjoy the programme just as much. There is no need to turn into a celebrity chef to enjoy the Water Detox. If you are eating out, just read through the list before you leave the house and then choose from the menu accordingly. You will be surprised at how easy it is to follow the programme in even the most expensive or basic restaurants, or even in sandwich bars. If you really are stuck, then start the trend of ordering 'off menu'. Ask if the chef can provide you with a combination that suits and see them rise to the challenge. If the rich and famous can do it, then I think we should give it a go too!

It is likely that you are one of the millions of people who follow a very similar routine every day of their lives. If you are not detoxing, it's extremely likely that you will have something like toast for breakfast, a sandwich, salad, soup or jacket potato for lunch and then an evening meal almost always consisting of pasta or potatoes, fish or meat, with vegetables. If you are eating out, this diet may vary a bit because someone else is doing the cooking. Or if you are away from home, it can change. But for the most part, what you eat each day will be very similar, day in, day out.

You can eat quite simply on the programme. Just choose the foods you like best and that are easiest for you, and stick to those foods throughout the 18 days. Do remember to read the lists fully, as you can then broaden your choice when you're eating out or entertaining without 'coming off' the Water Detox programme.

Alternatively, following the programme may give you the excuse to try out lots of different foods and meals. Experimentation can be good fun, and you may just stumble across a meal that eventually becomes one of your normal 'routine' meals, even when you are not detoxing!

Breakfasts

The old adage 'We should breakfast like kings, lunch like princes and dine like paupers' isn't far wrong. Although it is not strictly true on the Water Detox, the main meals or the bulk of the food you consume should be eaten during the day and certainly not late in the evening. When we have breakfast, it is the longest time our bodies have gone without food throughout the day: we have been asleep for approximately 8 hours, and we ate around 3 hours before that. Having a good breakfast is key to getting the body awake, full of energy and rehydrated after your night's sleep.

Juices and smoothies

If you have a juicer, the following recipes may just make your day.

Breakfast Pick-me-up

1 carrot	1 teaspoon grated ginger
1 apple	Juice of 1 lime
2 celery sticks	

Feed the carrot and the apple into the juicer, follow with the celery and then add the ginger. Mix in the juice of the lime and stir thoroughly. Drink as a wake-up call.

St Clement's

1 orange, peeled	1 apple
1 lemon, peeled	1 pear

Juice the orange, lemon, apple and pear. Drink up and owe me 5 farthings.

Grapeful

Handful each green and red grapes
1 small cube fresh ginger
2 apples

Juice all the ingredients and refresh your system.

Banana Breakfast

1 banana
1 dessertspoon of honey

1 slice honeydew melon –
   about a quarter of a small one
1 small pot sheep's yoghurt

Mix the banana and the honey together in a liquidiser or blender. Add the melon in cubes and then the yoghurt until the texture is as smooth as you want.

Watermelon Wake-up

Large slice of watermelon cut into pieces
   to fit into the juicer – quarter or half
   of a melon depending on its size and
   your hunger

1 small slice peeled ginger
Handful seedless black grapes

Juice and feel the flow.

Heartier options

Grilled Kippers and Tomatoes

Smoked kipper fillet
1 large beef tomato
Twist black pepper

A typical breakfast, but also totally detox. Slice the tomato and sprinkle with pepper. Serve with the fish and enjoy.

Feta and Watermelon

1 slice watermelon – quarter or a half,
    depending on size
50 g (2 oz) feta cheese

Cube the watermelon and place in a bowl. Cube the feta into the same size and mix together. Breakfast like a king.

Muesli

1 small pot sheep's yoghurt
1 teaspoon sunflower seeds
1 teaspoon sesame seeds
1 teaspoon pumpkin seeds
1 dessertspoon blueberries or blackberries

Pour the yoghurt into a bowl and mix in the seeds and fruit to taste. If you like runny yoghurt, just add more. If you like a thicker mixture, one pot should be enough.

Grilled Pineapple and Honey

Several hoops of pineapple
1 teaspoon honey
1 tablespoon goat's yoghurt (optional)

Place the pineapple hoops on a baking tray or ovenproof dish. Smooth the teaspoon of honey over the top, then place under a hot grill. Watch as the honey caramelises, then remove the pineapple. Serve with a tablespoon of yoghurt if desired.

Fruit Salad

Take a dessert bowl and fill with a mixture of your favourite fruits: blueberries, cherries, cranberries, dried or fresh or a combination of both.

Juice of 1 lime
1 dessertspoon honey

Mix the lime juice with the honey to make a runny syrup. Mix together the fruits and pour the honey blend over them. Stir gently so that the fruits and juices are coated with the syrup.

Snacks

Before we get down to the nitty-gritty of lunch and dinner, a word on snacks. We have already read about the fact that 75 per cent of our hunger pangs are actually requests from our body for water. So each time you feel hungry, have a glass of water. If you are still peckish 20 minutes later, you can have something to eat. Remember that the Water Detox is not a diet, but a healthy way to wash through and cleanse your body. If you are trying to lose weight, though, following the Water Detox will do this for you.

You shouldn't get hungry during the programme if you follow the guidelines of eating 5 smaller meals rather than 3 larger ones. But we are all human, and the need to snack is a great one! Choose any of the following to fill the gap and to stop you grabbing something to eat that is not totally detox.

Yoghurt

Mid-morning or mid-afternoon, a good way to fill up and keep it healthy is to have a pot of natural sheep's or goat's yoghurt. If you wish to enhance the flavour and add even more nutrition, stir in a teaspoon of honey of your choice. Yoghurt is 50 per cent water.

Crudités

There is nothing to stop you chopping up some vegetables and taking those to work or out with you in your bag. Better still, don't bother with chopping – carrots are excellent for crunching and you can buy them ready washed in most food shops. Chopped-up peppers and celery sticks will also keep hunger at bay and water flowing freely through your system.

Teas and tisanes

Drinking a large cup of herbal tea or just hot water can help make you feel full, and definitely add to your Water Detox. We often make a hot drink purely as a diversion when we've been talking to someone, or as a break when working. Usually we're making tea or coffee. On the Water Detox, simply do exactly the same as before, but make sure your refreshing or relaxing drink is caffeine-free this time. Remember: we can often feel hungry when we are actually thirsty, so try water or herbal teas to calm your hunger pangs and rehydrate at the same time. For more on tea, see page 71–4.

Hummus

I keep on about this snack, but it really is very useful to have around as it is very healthy. Chickpeas are over 50 per cent water, and it is great as a dip for crudités to make a more satisfying snack.

200 g (8 oz) chickpeas – either tinned, or fresh, soaked and cooked
3 fresh garlic cloves, peeled and crushed
3 tablespoons sesame seed paste (tahini)
Juice of 1 lemon
Juice of 1 lime
2 tablespoons olive oil or sesame seed oil
Pinch cayenne pepper and pinch paprika
Water

Put the chickpeas in a bowl and mash them into a smooth paste. If you want your hummus to be quite chunky, you just mash them to the consistency you require. Add the remaining ingredients one by one and mix continuously as you go. Once you have made a thick paste, you can add water slowly until it forms a thick creamy sauce.

Fruits

Eating any fruits from the list can serve as something to snack on. Make sure you don't eat much fruit after a meal; just eat it between meals to keep your hunger at bay.

Leftovers

If you have prepared a meal for your Water Detox programme and found that there is too much to manage – you will be eating slowly so you will be fully aware of how full you are from now on – you may find that you are cooking and preparing more than you need. As the Water Detox requires you to eat fresh, raw foods or to prepare foods freshly, you can be assured that there will be plenty of nutrition for the day after. If you cannot finish a meal then simply place it in a sealable container and store in the fridge. This will almost certainly serve as a great snack or filler for the following day. There really is no excuse for throwing food away. Waste not!

Lunches and Dinners

Remember that it is better to have 4 or 5 light meals a day than to sit down to a huge plate of food 3 times a day. Eating just 3 meals a day often causes big surges and drops in energy and blood sugar. This is more likely to have you reaching for something to satisfy your hunger that is not detox. 'Little and often' will keep you on the straight and narrow. The following recipes are designed to fill you up but not to overfill. You can, of course, adjust the amounts to suit your taste and as they are so delicious you will probably serve them to friends and family as well. Each recipe is for one person, so just multiply the amount by the number of guests you are expecting or family members you are feeding.

You can also serve some of the meals exactly as they are described or you could add some fish or other vegetables to boost or add courses.

Jacket Potatoes

Jacket potatoes are great for the Water Detox programme. You can basically add any of the vegetables from the list or any of the fish or cheeses and end up with quite a hearty meal.

You can also easily get jacket potatoes from snack or sandwich bars. As wheat doesn't feature in the H$_2$O Nutrition Programme, you can almost think of your potato as the alternative to the sandwich. Just don't think that potatoes can form the mainstay of every meal. They may be over 70 per cent water, but they should be eaten in moderation.

Filling suggestions for your potatoes

Hummus and tomatoes

Flaked tuna and feta

Watercress, feta and beetroot – my personal favourite (drizzle a little oil and half a lemon over it, and it's just what the doctor ordered)

Roquefort and walnuts

Green salad

Mushrooms

Homemade ratatouille

Roast garlic

Grilled salmon fillet

And just about anything else from the lists that you imagination allows ... that you imagination allows ...

Green Soup

Half an onion

3 or 4 garlic cloves

Quarter of a medium green cabbage – Savoy is good

250 ml (1/2 pint) vegetable stock

Olive oil

1 large potato

1 teacup wild rice

Black pepper

Finely chop the onion, garlic and cabbage. Heat a teaspoon of olive oil in a pan. Lightly stir fry the onion and garlic until transparent and going golden brown. Add the cabbage and keep over the heat until it becomes softer and brighter in colour. Remove from the heat and put to one side.

Chop the potato into 1 cm cubes and add to the stock. Boil until the potato is soft. Add the rice and keep cooking until the rice is tender. Add the rice, stock and potatoes to the cabbage, garlic and onions. Stir so that all the ingredients are mixed together and then season with black pepper to taste. Take a quarter of the soup and blend to a smooth creamy texture. Add this blend back to the main pan and stir again. This should make the soup creamy, but hearty and chunky. Serve.

Pumpkin Soup

1 medium pumpkin	Brown rice
1 large onion, chopped	Water
500 ml (1 pint) vegetable stock	Sheep's yoghurt
Thyme and bay leaves	Paprika and pepper, to taste

Scoop out, or peel and cut up, the flesh from the pumpkin and put in a pan together with the chopped onion, stock and the herbs. Boil for 20 minutes or until the pumpkin is tender. Pour off the remaining stock but don't throw it away. Cook the brown rice in water until tender. Drain. Take the herbs out of the pumpkin and onion mix, and using a blender, food processor or mashing tool, mash the pumpkin to a creamy consistency. Add the rice to the pumpkin mixture, and then, in a pan, slowly add the reserved stock while heating the mix until you have a smooth rice and pumpkin soup.

To serve, spoon a dollop of yoghurt onto the top and swirl around. Season with paprika and pepper to taste.

Tomato Gazpacho

4 large tomatoes, chopped, or 1 large tin	Juice of 1 lime
1 small red pepper	1 tablespoon olive oil
1 small cooked beetroot	Freshly ground black pepper
2 fresh garlic cloves	1 dessertspoon sheep's yoghurt
Juice of 1 lemon	

Place all the ingredients except for the yoghurt in a blender and blend until everything is well mixed and red in colour. You can carry on blending if you like smooth soups, or leave it chunky if you like more texture to your meal. Chill the soup for at least an hour in the fridge, then serve in a bowl, with the yoghurt lightly stirred in.

Red Rice Salad

Two large tablespoons uncooked red rice
Olive oil
2 shallots or 1 medium red onion, chopped or diced
Black pepper
1 fresh lime
1 tablespoon crumbled feta cheese
2 or 3 sprigs fresh coriander, finely chopped

Cook the rice following the instructions on the packet. Put a teaspoon of olive oil into a frying pan and fry the shallots or onions until slightly soft and browned at the edges. Add the cooked rice to the onions in the pan and stir to absorb the flavour of the onions in the oil. Add 3 or 4 grinds of black pepper and squeeze the juice of the fresh lime into the pan. Transfer the rice and onions to a plate and sprinkle the feta cheese and coriander over the top.

Stir Fried Rice

100 g (4 oz) brown rice
1 large tablespoon peas
1 onion
1 carrot
3 spring onions
Olive oil
¼ cucumber
1 salmon fillet
Soy sauce

Boil the brown rice until tender, adding the peas for the last 8 minutes of the cooking. Drain the pea and rice mix. Slice the onion, carrot and spring onions into very thin strips. Lightly stir fry these vegetables in the olive oil until just tender. Slice the cucumber into thin strips and add to the vegetables, then remove from the heat. Grill the salmon until cooked through but not dry. Allow the fish to cool and then flake. Put all the ingredients together, rice and peas, vegetables and cucumber, and the fish. Mix lightly. Season with a few splashes of soy sauce and serve while still hot.

Rainbow Rice

Cherry tomatoes
Yellow and orange peppers
Beetroot, cooked
Courgettes

Fresh coriander
Short grain brown rice
Olive oil
Lime juice

The above amounts are to taste, or depend on how hungry you are.

This salad can be made as raw as possible – except the rice of course! Chop the tomatoes in half. Cut the orange and yellow peppers lengthways into thin strips. Cube the cooked beetroot, then slice the courgettes into long, thick ribbons. Finely chop the coriander. Boil the rice until tender.

Using a griddle pan, grill the courgettes. They will take on a striped appearance from the griddle pan. Mix the coriander and all the vegetables, except the courgettes, into the boiled rice. Put on a plate, then place the grilled courgette ribbons over the top. Drizzle a teaspoon of olive oil over the top, followed by the lime juice.

Wild Rice and Salsa

Red onion
2 garlic cloves
Olive oil
Cooked wild rice
Cooked kidney beans, or use tinned
Spring onions
Chilli pepper

Red peppers
Green peppers
Passionfruit
Fresh coriander
Lime juice
Black pepper

The above amounts are to taste, or depend on how hungry you are.

Chop the red onion and the garlic. Fry in a teaspoon of olive oil until the onion is caramelised. Add the rice and kidney beans and continue to fry lightly until all ingredients have blended together and are coated in the juices.

To make the salsa, chop the spring onions, chilli pepper, and red and green peppers into very small cubes or slivers. Scoop out the passionfruit and add to the chopped vegetables. Chop the coriander and blend into the salsa mix. Add the juice of a lime, a little olive oil and some black pepper. Stir everything together.

Put the rice and kidney beans on a plate. Add a large spoonful of the salsa mix, and get on down!

Detox Paella

Shallots	Fish stock
Olive oil	3 small fillets oily fish, preferably of
Peppers	different types – salmon, herring,
Courgettes	mackerel, whitebait, tuna …
Broad beans	Tomatoes
Long grain rice	Parsley

The above amounts are to taste, or depend on how hungry you are.

Slice the shallots and lightly fry in the olive oil. Chop the peppers and courgettes into strips. Add these with the broad beans to the shallot mix and stir together. Add the rice and stir around until coated with juices from the vegetables, then add the stock. Boil until nearly tender, adding more stock if needed, but don't overcook the rice. Once the rice is nearly done, add the pieces of fish and continue to cook until they have gone opaque. Make sure the fish is totally cooked before serving. Slice the tomatoes and finely chop the parsley and scatter over the top before serving.

You may steam or grill the fish and serve on top of the Detox Paella if you prefer.

New Potato Salad with Beans and Peas

5 or 6 new potatoes	Cucumber
French green beans	Spring onions
Mangetout	Yoghurt
Peas	Lemon juice
Green pepper	Olive oil

The above amounts are to taste, or depend on how hungry you are.

Boil the potatoes until tender. Steam the green beans, mangetout and peas until tender. Chop the green pepper into small cubes and stir fry until slightly brown. Chop the cucumber and spring onions and mix into the yoghurt.

Slice all the potatoes in half and mix with the peppers, peas and beans. Pour over the lemon juice and olive oil, and toss together so that they are coated in the dressing. Spoon the yoghurt mix on top of the vegetables and tuck in.

Hot Grilled Cabbage

Half a small cabbage – red is preferable	Soft goat's cheese
Half a red onion	Cayenne pepper
1 tablespoon cooked wild rice	

Slice the red cabbage and stir fry so that it is still crunchy. Or you can steam or boil it – whichever is your preferred method. Fry the chopped red onion so that it is translucent and still crunchy, then add the cabbage and put in a serving bowl. Top with the wild rice, then break the soft cheese over the top and sprinkle lightly with cayenne pepper. Grill so that the cheese is toasted on top but not burnt.

Garlic and Ginger Vegetables with Goat's or Sheep's Cheese

Large portion mixed carrots, broccoli, and shredded cabbage – red or green
4 tablespoons water
1 teaspoon crushed ginger
2 fresh garlic cloves, finely chopped
1 tablespoon grated hard goat's or sheep's cheese
Small sprig coriander, finely chopped

Cut the vegetables into narrow strips. Place in a large dish and mix in the water, ginger and garlic, and sprinkle the cheese over the top. Bake at 180°C/350°F/Gas 4 for about 50 minutes or until the vegetables are tender. Serve with more fresh ginger and coriander sprinkled on top.

Garlic Crush

1 medium garlic bulb
1 large jacket potato, sliced in wedges and baked
Olive oil
Lemon juice, to taste
A good friend

This is served in many restaurants as a starter. The potato wedges can be replaced by crusty bread.

Take the whole bulb of garlic and roast in a hot oven for 30 minutes. Check that it is cooked through by seeing if the individual cloves are soft when you squeeze them.

Serve the garlic bulb on a small side plate and simply squeeze the contents of each clove onto a potato wedge, spread it over, and tuck in. For extra nutrients you can drizzle over a little olive oil and a squeeze of lemon juice. Share this meal with a friend so that at least two of you smell fresh and healthy!

Oven-baked Stuffed Vegetables

For this recipe you can choose the vegetable you want to stuff. You can do beef tomatoes – the very large ones – marrows, peppers or courgettes. Sometimes you can get wonderful round courgettes such as patty pan. These are easier to manage than the long, thin variety.

1 large vegetable of choice	Seedless grapes, red or green, sliced
1 red onion, chopped	Olive oil
1 finely sliced garlic clove	Creamed/soft goat's cheese
Cooked brown rice	Watercress dressed with olive oil and
Handful chopped basil leaves	lemon

Hollow out the vegetable you are going to stuff and place on a baking tray in a medium oven (180°C/350°F/Gas 4) for 10 minutes to soften. Lightly stir fry the onion and garlic. Mix in the cooked brown rice, the chopped basil and the sliced grapes. Stuff the vegetable with this mix, drizzle olive oil over, and place a slice of the goat's cheese on top. Bake in the oven for a further 10 minutes or until ready.

Serve with a large handful of watercress with olive oil and lemon juice dressing. Be careful when you tuck into the stuffed vegetable. The grapes are so full of water that they may be extremely hot to handle!

Beans and Herbs

5 or 6 spring onions, topped and tailed and split at the green end down the middle	Sprigs of dill, parsley and coriander
	Sunflower oil
	Juice of 1 lemon
Large handful fresh broad beans	Freshly ground black pepper
2 or 3 broccoli florets	Soft sheep's cheese
Quarter of a fennel bulb, finely chopped	

Take a bowl of iced water and drop in the spring onions – the ends should curl if the water is cold enough. Remove from the water once they have curled over. Mix together the beans, onions, broccoli, and fennel and put on a plate. Chop the herbs or rip the leaves and sprinkle over the bean mix. Drizzle the oil over the salad to taste, then squeeze the lemon onto the plate through your hands so that the pips stay off the plate. Grind the black pepper and crumble the cheese over the top. You can either serve the dish cool and fresh or place the plate under the grill for a couple of minutes until the cheese begins to brown and melt.

Yoghurt Dip

Take any of the vegetables from the list on page 42 that you wish, enough to fill a serving plate, to make crudités. Cooked jacket potato wedges make good dippers, too.

1 pot sheep's yoghurt
1 small onion, finely diced
1 garlic clove, finely diced

Juice of 1 lemon
1 handful watercress and coriander, chopped into very fine flakes

Chop the vegetables into bite-size crudités. Mix the yoghurt with the onion, garlic, lemon juice and herbs and place in a small serving bowl. Dip the vegetables and/or potato wedges into the yoghurt dip and enjoy.

Pear, Walnut and Rocket Salad with Roquefort

1 pear
Handful walnut kernels
Large handful of rocket leaves

50 g (2 oz) Roquefort, crumbled or cubed
1 tablespoon walnut oil
Balsamic vinegar

Slice the pear into eighths, removing the core and stem. Holding the walnut kernels in your hand over a bowl, squeeze them together to crush them lightly. Wash the rocket and place on a plate. Fan out the pear slices on the rocket, then sprinkle the walnut pieces over. Crumble the Roquefort or scatter it in cubes over the top, then drizzle both the walnut oil and balsamic vinegar over everything. Serve.

Nut Salad

2 tablespoons cashew nuts
2 tablespoons pine nuts
1 cooked beetroot, shredded or sliced
Shredded watercress
2 tablespoons chopped fresh coriander
    leaves

Grated carrot
4 tablespoons nut or olive oil
Juice of 1/2 lemon
Poppy seeds

Toss all the ingredients together and serve. Alternatively, you can serve this mixture on a bed of brown rice or as an accompaniment to any of the main course dishes.

Mango Salad

White fish fillet of your choice
Long grain red rice
Vegetable stock
1 large mango
Small cherry tomatoes
Pistachio nuts

Coriander leaves
Mild chilli pepper
Chopped mint leaves
Red pepper
Lime juice

The above amounts are to taste, or depend on how hungry you are.

Grill the fish. Boil the rice in vegetable stock until tender but not soggy. Chop the mango, tomatoes and nuts into small cubes and finely chop the herbs and spices, making sure to keep all the fruit and tomato juices. They will keep the rice moist for the raw ingredients. When the fish is cool, flake it.

Mix the raw fruit and vegetables into the rice, then stir in the flaked fish. Pour over the juice of the lime and the reserved juice of the mango and tomatoes. Taste, season with black pepper if required, and serve.

Beetroot and Tzatziki

1 large fresh beetroot	1 garlic clove
Olive oil	Cucumber
Lemon juice	Yoghurt – sheep's or goat's
Freshly ground black pepper	Sea salt

Boil the beetroot until tender – approximately 25 minutes for medium, 45 for large. Peel and slice the beetroot and fan out on a plate. Pour over the olive oil and lemon juice and season with freshly ground black pepper. To make the tzatziki, crush the garlic and finely crush the cucumber, then mix into the yoghurt and add a little sea salt to taste.

Dip the beetroot into the creamy, rich yoghurt dressing and enjoy.

Roast Broccoli with Tuna

1 tablespoon brown rice	1 teaspoon toasted shredded
almonds	Juice of 1 whole lime
Olive oil	1 tablespoon coriander, chopped
1 large flower broccoli, split into florets	Black pepper
1 fillet/portion cooked fresh tuna, tuna	
strips or tinned tuna in spring water	

While boiling the rice, place a roasting tray with a tablespoon of olive oil in the bottom of it in a hot 220°C/425°F/Gas 7 oven. When the oil is hot, place the broccoli florets on the roasting tray, roast for 5 minutes, then turn and continue to roast until they are slightly browned and soft in the middle. Take the cooked tuna and flake. When the rice is cooked, mix with the flaked tuna and the almonds. Toss with the lime juice, a teaspoon of olive oil and chopped coriander, and place on a dinner plate. Lay the cooked broccoli on the bed of rice and tuna, and serve with a twist of fresh black pepper.

Tuna Rice

1 small tin or medium fillet of tuna
Olive oil
1 heaped tablespoon of cooked
  rice

1 tablespoon red kidney beans, cooked
  or tinned
2 small beetroots, cooked or pickled
Balsamic vinegar

If using fresh tuna, brush with olive oil and grill. Flake the tuna and mix in with the rice and kidney beans. Dice the beetroot and sprinkle on top of the tuna/rice/bean mix. Pour 2 teaspoons of olive oil and balsamic vinegar dressing over the fish mix.

Steamed Fish with Ginger

White fish fillet of your choice
Sesame oil
Grated fresh ginger slivers, or
  minced ginger from a jar

Spring onions
Sesame seeds

Place the fish in a steamer, or if you don't have one you can wrap the fish in foil and use a colander over a pan of boiling water. Before closing the wrapping, put a teaspoon of sesame oil on the fish and place a sliver of ginger both under and on top of the fish. Strew chopped-up spring onions and sesame seeds over, then close the parcel and steam for 10 to 15 minutes.

Be careful when you open the parcel, as the steam will rush out and could burn your fingers or face. Stand well back!

Grilled Sardines

2 or 3 fresh sardines
Olive oil

Lettuce of your choice
1 lemon, cut into quarters

Brush the sardines with the oil and grill until wonderfully crispy. Place on a large plate of assorted lettuce of your choice, then drizzle on the remaining olive oil, squeeze the lemon juice over and tuck in.

Salmon and Tarragon

1 salmon fillet
1 dessertspoon tarragon leaves, chopped
Handful of watercress on the stem
2 tablespoons cooked brown rice

1 teaspoon honey
1 teaspoon sunflower oil
Juice of 1 lime

Grill the salmon fillet until pink and tender. Chop the tarragon and watercress and mix into the brown rice. Put the honey, oil and lime juice into a cup and stir together or shake together in a jar. Put the rice on a serving plate. Place the salmon fillet on top, and pour over the dressing.

Fresh Fish Ceviche

This recipe requires very fresh fish fillets but is superb, simple, very healthy, and wonderful for entertaining. Just make sure your fishmonger knows the fish is going to be served 'raw'.

Fish fillet of your choice
Juice of 2 fresh limes
Fresh parsley – flatleaf is good

Oil to drizzle
Black pepper

Cut the fresh fish into thin strips and marinade in the lime juice for at least 2 hours. Make sure the fish is covered with the juice or it won't 'turn'. Put the parsley in a cup and chop it very fine with some scissors.

You will know if the fish is ready if it has turned opaque. Place the strips on a plate and sprinkle the parsley over the top. Drizzle on the oil to taste and sprinkle with black pepper.

Grilled Tuna with Anchovy Lattice

Tuna fillet

2 or 3 anchovy pieces

Cherry tomatoes or larger tomatoes, chopped into very small pieces

Olive oil

Red onion, in hoops or finely chopped

Coriander

Grill the tuna until cooked through, with a little pink remaining in the centre. Thinly slice the anchovy fillets into very thin strips.

Crisscross the anchovy fillets on the tuna fillet and place a small piece of cherry tomato in between each 'diamond' of the lattice. Drizzle a little oil over the fish and serve with raw red onion and chopped coriander.

Desserts

Just because you are detoxing doesn't mean you cannot have healthy helpings of pudding. Remember to keep most fruits for the start of the meal, as they are more easily digested on an empty stomach, and then you can keep cheese for the end of the meal. Some of the most delicious cheeses can be at their best when eaten simply with celery or grapes.

Cheese and Celery Plate

Use chevre, Roquefort, feta, manchego or any other goat's or sheep's cheese available from the supermarket or cheesemongers. Keep the slices very thin as you don't want to have too much concentrated fats.

Celery sticks

Grapes, red or green

Place a selection of three cheeses on a plate and garnish with celery and grapes. You do not need biscuits with the cheese. You can simply eat it with the help of a knife and fork or your fingers. You may feel you're actually tasting the cheeses for the first time.

Honey Nut 'Soups'

1 pot yoghurt
1 teaspoon honey
Handful almonds or nuts of your choice

Lightly mix or totally blend the yoghurt together with the honey. Sprinkle the nuts into the blend. Serve chilled.

SOMETHING TO DRINK?

When you are following the Water Detox programme, remember to avoid drinking with food. It prevents the full absorption of essential nutrients and can upset the digestive process. Drink half an hour before and you may find you are not as hungry as you thought and then wait until at least an hour after eating to have your next drink. The foods you are eating are so high in water content that you should not get thirsty. If you are, check your foods and get more vegetables on the plate.

The Tea Ceremony

One of the first questions that people ask me when we talk about detoxing is 'Do I have to give up coffee and alcohol?' Even just the idea of giving up these substances puts people into mild panic. I can eat healthily, but if you ask me to give up the two things I rely on then it would be totally out of the question. And I am up there with the rest of you when it comes to giving up either my Friday evening glass of red or my early morning coffee. It would be a total nightmare! The good thing is that it used to be my Friday evening half bottle (if I was good) of red and my daily 6 or 7 cups of coffee. Then I did the 30-Day Detox Yourself programme and my routine is now a fresh coffee at around 9.30 a.m. and an evening red wine intake of 1 or 2 glasses. The fact is, I now really taste the coffee, and instant tastes pretty yukky, stale and fake, so I don't ask for coffee any more. And the wine seems

71

to have a good flavour and effect even after the first glass, so 2 is about my maximum in any normal situation. There are times, and my friends will prove this, when I can have a good time like the rest of you, but as a rule I don't need to drink anywhere near as much as I used to.

The 30-Day Detox Yourself programme meant that giving them both up made me realise how much was 'wasted' and not doing me any good. The coffee I was drinking was horrible, and I was quite happy downing that first glass of wine without even tasting it properly or taking the time to enjoy the flavour. After the detox, my body felt so clean and my taste buds were once more so alive that I could still be just as satisfied – but with a fifth of the amount. It not only saved my health, it also had a decent impact on my budget.

Which brings me to tea. Now, it is perfectly true to say that tea has the same amount of caffeine as coffee, but that we use less tea to make a cup than we do coffee. But ordinary, caffeinated tea is not what we are talking about. We are talking about green and herbal teas. These are not only extremely good for us; they also come in an amazing array of flavours, and specific uses.

Green tea is full of flavonoids. Flavonoids are chemical compounds that are generally believed to be antioxidant, antibacterial, anti-inflammatory and all-round health enhancers and improvers. The more you include in your diet, the more you are doing for your body.

Drinking flavonoid-packed green tea is best. Green jasmine and Oolong are very good, and Indian, Earl Grey and Ceylon black teas are still pretty good in terms of flavonoids. Drunk in moderation, all these teas will build your body's ability to fight free radicals and toxins.

Decrease the caffeine and/or stimulant content by steeping the tea in hot water briefly, then throwing away the first 'brew' and adding more water. Drinking one good cup of tea a day will hydrate and protect you.

If tea doesn't appeal, try herbal teas or tisanes. They are more or less the same but 'tisane' is sometimes used to refer to herbal teas made with the fresh leaf of the plant or herb, rather than the dried and bagged herb.

The first time I had a tisane was in Chile. We had finished a lovely meal and then I was offered tea. I accepted it, as they had promised me it was really good and a great digestif after the spicy food we had just eaten.

The tea arrived. It was a beautiful fresh green colour and smelled amazing. The only problem in identifying it was my inability to conquer even the most basic understanding of Spanish – not to mention the nuances of the Chilean variety. I now have sufficient Spanish to identify and discover the secret of this amazing tea on my next trip. I just hope it was legal!

Peppermint
Digestive and very stimulating.

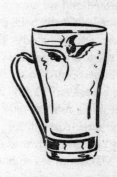

Maté
Refreshing and balancing, oxygenating.

Bergamot
Relaxing.

Raspberry leaf
Full of vitamin C and also good for preparing the womb for birth – not an everyday occurrence, I know, but worth knowing all the same if you become pregnant. (No detox is advised for pregnant or nursing women.)

Ginseng
Stimulates the brain; balancing and purging.

Chamomile
Relaxing, digestive, settles the stomach.

Ginger
Digestive and stimulating, very cleansing.

There are hundreds more teas available. A favourite combination of mine is ginseng with jasmine. I find ginseng tea on its own too dry and 'chewy', but add the jasmine and I cannot get enough of it. It is worth persevering with teas until you find a favourite. The secret is to discover one that you find really delicious. As soon as this happens you have almost certainly solved the problem of how to get used to your 2 litres per day as well as how to give up caffeinated hot drinks – tea, coffee, and so on.

Earlier in this chapter I mentioned that one of the main reasons why we drink caffeine is that it is a ritual we have which marks a well-earned break. If we have reached the point in the day where one job is finished and we are starting another, one phone call that needed to be made has finally been made, a desk that needed to be tidied can finally been seen through the paperwork, or a playroom carpet reappears after all the toys are put away – then a cup of tea is our reward. Don't change a thing: reward yourself, but make sure your hot drink is fresh and of the herbal variety. Boil the kettle, sit down with the warm mug and feel the water refresh, relax, invigorate and concentrate the mind for the next task. You will find yourself fully prepared and hydrated, without any chemical downside.

Make your tea an hourly ritual that keeps your fluid levels high, and cleanses and stimulates naturally and continually. But remember also that your tea is on top of your 2-litre requirement.

3

Hydrotherapy

THE USE OF WATER IN therapeutic treatments can advance the body's healing capacity immensely. During the 18-day programme you are asked to introduce a minimum of 3 such treatments. You can do more. In fact, I think you will almost certainly do more, but try to make sure you introduce 3 new ones alongside the familiar favourites.

- Kneipp bathing

- Sauna and steam

- Jacuzzi and hot tub

- Colonic irrigation

- Walking by the sea

- Watsu

- Swimming with dolphins

- Bathing

- Cool showers

A BRIEF HISTORY OF BATHING

The Greeks, Romans and Turks are all well known for their love affair with bathing. In today's Turkish baths, or hammams, you can still spend the day in a steamy atmosphere having the toxins purged from your body. The experience is great, and the massage some of the deepest you can find.

The original aim of bathing was for total indulgence. Cleanliness was rare, so the bathing rituals of the wealthy were indulgence indeed. From these early times, taking the waters was combined with massage, and cold and hot water application – the very first detoxification spas in history.

The Japanese use bathing as a ritual. Some of the most amazing baths you can find are the huge wooden Japanese troughs that whole groups would wallow in for hours.

The Scandanavians are famous for their bathing habits – small wooden huts, heated saunas, steam, birch-twig switches and rolling in the snow. Back in England we have spa towns such as Bath and Leamington Spa, France has the world-famous town of Vichy and Germany boasts Baden Baden.

Visiting spas is still popular as a way to indulge in treatments using water to heal our tired and stressed bodies. But you don't need to book a flight to benefit from the same treatments. Simply read on and bring the spa to your own home: bathing has never been so simple.

If you think of all the treatments that you can have at a spa or salon that involve pure water, it soon becomes clear that water is an integral aspect of our 'therapy' treatments. Flotation, hot tubs, jacuzzis, jet showers, plunge pools, Turkish baths, swimming, sitz baths, blitz showers, bucket plunge, Vichy showers – the list goes on and on. Not only does every treatment involve water, but more importantly, every treatment involves different temperatures of water, or alternating temperatures of water within the same treatment. This technique is known as hydrotherapy. Don't forget that every treatment will also involve the resonance and the vibration of the particular water used. It is not just wet, it is positively charged with nutrients and goodies ... 'I'm picking up good vibrations' ...

Then there are the many treatments that involve water but not immersion in it – steam, inhalations, vapours, wraps and packs. And lots of extremely beneficial treatments or therapies use water as the 'agent' to facilitate the treatment. These include Watsu, flotation, colonic irrigation, flushing, flower essences and homeopathic remedies.

During the Water Detox you will get the opportunity to indulge in or experience at least 6 treatments – 3 thalassotherapy and 3 hydrotherapy – and then you can add in skin and body care. I discuss thalassotherapy in Chapter 4. Below is the lowdown on hydrotherapy. Hopefully it will give you a better understanding of those treatments you have never heard of, introduce some totally new treatments into your life and explain away some of the myths about the others.

USING FLOWING WATER

Hydrotherapy is the term given to treatments or therapies using water in its flowing state. It can mean using spring or natural mineral waters, but in any case water is the key ingredient. And temperature is the key characteristic.

Hydrotherapy uses water at varying temperatures, and it is this aspect that is the most effective or therapeutic. Applying hot and cold water during the same treatment is extremely beneficial if not crucial. In hydrotherapy, the application of hot and cold water during a treatment is known as 'short-term' application. This helps the body to work at optimum levels: the application of hot and cold at the right temperatures and for the right period of time means that the body can concentrate on cleansing, rejuvenation and repair. If we get it wrong and apply hot or cold water for too long, the body needs to stop the 'repair' process and move into 'protect and survive'. Getting the balance of application right is essential.

As we all know, bathing in hot water is simply wonderful. Getting into a warm bath and relaxing for a while can do no end of good. But imagine being in the hot bath and instead of the water slowly cooling and you getting out of the bath when you have had enough, you are asked to stay in the water at the same temperature it was when you started – nice and hot. Pretty soon you might begin to feel a bit too hot, like you are overheating, or you may even feel faint and in need of some air or at least cooling of some sort. It doesn't make the relaxing bath seem nice any more; in fact it begins to seem quite claustrophobic.

Here's another way of thinking about it. Snuggling under a duvet on a cold night is a lovely, relaxing experience. But what if you woke in the middle of the night feeling far too hot? The once-comforting duvet has now become an overheating machine and you need to immediately kick it off or stick an arm or a leg out of the bed to cool down. Yet you are unable to and you have to stay where you are, all tucked in. You will experience the same feelings of overheating and fainting.

The upshot of all this is that your body cannot tolerate high temperatures for too long a period of time. Once it becomes too warm, it will attempt to cool down. It will send blood away from the centre of the body and out to the extremities so that it cools down and doesn't 'cook' our internal organs. The long-term application of heat will cause the body to go into protection mode – not very relaxing or therapeutic.

So with heat, it's all in the timing. Incredibly relaxing and therapeutic in the short term – and we will go on to see just how remarkable the effects can be – to uncomfortable and depleting in the longer term.

It's a very similar story with the application of cold water. Short-term application can be wonderfully refreshing, but use it for too long and it becomes freezing and debilitating. Imagine: you go outside on a hot day to feel the cool, refreshing breeze on your face and arms. You cool down and feel balanced again. Now think how you would begin to feel if you are still sitting in that breeze a few minutes later: your arms get goose pimples and you begin to shiver. You have become too cold and the body doesn't like it any more. The body needs to protect itself, so just as with overheating, it begins shifting your blood supply, this time to the core organs to protect them and prevent them from cooling down to a dangerous and stagnating level.

We need to make sure we apply hydrotherapy treatments at the right temperatures and for the right length of time. The treatment should achieve the optimum benefits from alternating temperatures of water without triggering any of the body's negative 'protect and survive' mechanisms.

The actual effects of the short-term application of hot and cold are listed below. The benefits are really quite phenomenal and totally underestimated by most of us – no longer will a cold shower be a bad thing!

Here comes the science . . .

The Heat is On

The short-term effect of heat on the body is fabulously therapeutic. When we talk about 'short term', we are looking at anything between 5 and 15 minutes. It is entirely dependent on the individual and their body's tolerance to heat. Some people can stand the hottest summer day that the sun can throw at them, and some need to retire to the shade and the cool breezes after 5 minutes. Observing a 15-minute maximum ensures that the body is perfectly happy with the temperature while definitely benefiting from the therapeutic effects.

It is no coincidence that when we are ill, we 'get a temperature'. Although this is not short term, it does show that 'hothousing' the body will create an environment for the body to be able to fight illness, process germs, build immunity and get better sooner. Fever is the body's way of applying thermotherapy – alternating heat and cooling. When we have a fever we have periods of sweat and periods of shivers, the optimum environment for the body to process illness and recover. Hydrotherapy is the external application of thermotherapy through the use of water.

Here's what the application of heat can do.

• **Causes vasodilation** A widening of the blood vessels, which in turn increases the blood flow around the body. If we imagine that blood is the fuel for the body, the 'petrol' that keeps the body functioning at total efficiency, then we can see that increasing the blood flow and enabling it to pump more efficiently will benefit the whole body immediately and totally. It will flush out waste products and cleanse internal organs. Everything is boosted and on 'full flow'.

- **Increases circulation** If we have increased the blood flow around the body, then we have definitely increased circulation. We go to the gym to increase circulation after strenuous exercise. We know that increased circulation is fantastic for the body. It means that everything is being fully supplied with all the blood it needs for optimum operation. The organs are pumping, the skin is flushing and the body is cleansing and processing.

- **Increases metabolism** If our organs and systems are being supplied with optimum levels of blood through increased circulation, they can operate efficiently and perform their functions more efficiently. Our metabolism increases and improves the rate at which the body processes foods and therefore toxins.

- **Increases pulse rate** When we get hot, our pulse quickens and the heart pumps faster. A healthy heart can do this with no problem. But if you know you have heart disease, consult your doctor before using the application of heat.

- **Increases cell metabolism** The rate at which the body manufactures good chemicals such as hormones becomes more efficient or more balanced. This is a huge benefit of hydrotherapy.

- **Increases lymph function** As the body is heated, the blood pumps around the system and the tiny movements of the blood vessels improve the working function of the lymph system – our body's waste disposal system. This improves internal cleansing and elimination.

- **Decreases the stimulus of the myoneural junction** Our muscles and nerves are constantly in communication with each other. We move our legs forward when we think about walking, we sit up as soon as our brains hear the request and we go to catch a falling object without any conscious thought. It happens automatically as our nerves yell at the muscles to lurch forward. Application of heat slows this 'conversation' down and everything goes into deep relaxation and reduced response times. When relaxed, we move a lot more slowly. Heat relaxes the muscle response, and gives it a much-needed break.

- **Reduces spasticity in the muscles** Application of heat relaxes the muscles to the extent that we can do further work with the muscle fibres. It's like warming up before exercise to gain flexibility. We have a massage to warm our muscles before the deep work occurs in order to relax the tension and melt away the tightness. Application of heat allows increased range in movement, and reduced tension.

So overall, with the application of heat the body becomes deeply relaxed, recovers, and repairs takes place more efficiently. And the short-term application seems to give all these benefits almost immediately.

Use heat for longer than 15 minutes, though, and it becomes 'long-term' application, which depresses the circulatory system. Earlier I gave you a sketchy idea of what happens then, but here are the specifics. If you continue to apply heat, the body will take up to a third of blood away from the central organs and brain, to allow cooling. This means that the body will feel very relaxed or tired. Longer-term heat will make you feel uncomfortable, possibly claustrophobic, as you will have reduced the blood supply to key areas of the body to keep them cool. Dizziness could occur as blood is moved away from the brain.

Going for Cold

If the short-term application of heat relaxes, 2 to 5 minutes of cold applied to the body refreshes and invigorates. We all know just how startling it is to have a cold shower – and how great we feel afterwards.

The short-term application of cold has the following beneficial effects.

- **Causes vasoconstriction** Application of cold will constrict the blood vessels, a phenomenon known as vasoconstriction. The narrowing of blood vessels restricts blood supply to areas and in effect pushes blood away from an area that was previously flooded with blood.

- **Has an analgesic effect** The body releases a natural pain relief substance, prostaglandin, into muscle when cold is applied. This in turn reduces muscle spindle spasticity and gives relief from the painful cramps of muscle tension. It also means, in therapeutic terms, that the muscles won't hurt as much if they are being worked or manipulated if the area has been cooled down in some way.

- **Creates a beneficial 'shock' effect** When we experience the application of cold, water jets, cold showers, plunge pools and so on, one of the things that can be guaranteed is the deep inhalation of breath we take when it hits. We need to take that deep breath in order to catch our breath from the shock of cold water. This means we fully expand our lungs and therefore fully oxygenate our blood.

- **Prevents muscle damage** Necrosin is a natural chemical that destroys tissue when we damage a muscle. If you get the muscle cold as soon as it is damaged through, say, a hard workout or a deep tissue massage, the damage will be limited because cold inhibits the release of necrosin.

- **Reduces inflammation** When we have damaged or overused a muscle, it is likely to become inflamed. Inflammation restricts movement around the area of damage, in effect protecting it, but it can also lead to a build-up of scar tissue that can eventually restrict movement for good. Application of cold will reduce inflammation by making sure that excess blood is pushed away from the area, keeping the swelling down and manageable.

Short-term application of cold is extremely beneficial, but over the long term it can lead to stagnation and a dangerous restriction of blood supply to an area.

If you get the combination of hot and cold application just right, its therapeutic properties are unparalleled. Delivered incorrectly, it can be a mixture of hot and sweaty with cold and clammy, with no benefit except to check the body's ability to protect and survive instead of rebuilding and regenerating.

Hot and cold applied alternately also help balance acidity and alkalinity (pH) in the body.

The aim of hydrotherapy is to cause a 'rollercoaster' effect with the applications of hot and cold.

First
Heat is applied:

- Vasodilation

- Increased metabolism

- Increased pulse rate

- Increased circulation

- Increased cell metabolism

- Increased lymph function

- The body becomes deeply relaxed

- Healing takes place more efficiently

- The body eventually adjusts and homeostasis is reached

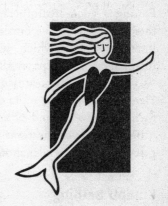

Then
Cold is applied:

- Immediate vasoconstriction

- Sharp intake of breath/oxygenation

- Analgesic effect

- Inhibits release of necrosin

- Reduction of inflammation

- The body pumps blood to the core organs to keep them warm and eventually adjusts so that homeostasis is reached.

Then heat is applied, etc . . .
Then cold is applied, etc . . .

If you rotate the application of hot and cold during the treatment over 5 to 15-minute periods, there will be a continuous process of vasoconstriction and vasodilation, which results in increased flushing rates within the body and optimum healing.

Heat and cold do more together than they can ever do apart

During a good hydrotherapy treatment or session, you should be totally relaxed on the outside while the body will be doing a heavy internal workout which will ultimately result in the body feeling totally relaxed both physically and emotionally.

There are many treatments involving water that can truly detoxify. Here are a few of the more common or readily available. Any or all of them are powerful and extremely effective. First we'll look at the ones using alternate applications of hot and cold water, then we'll investigate some of the wilder shores of hydrotherapy.

Kneipp Bathing

The 19th-century German Sebastian Kneipp was a great believer in the power and therapeutic qualities of water. He believed that the free flow of our blood and circulation was the secret to total health and wellbeing. Kneipp was one of the first practitioners to use the alternating temperatures of water to boost the body's circulation to gain optimum health.

We owe the wonderful sitz bath to Kneipp, the cold bathing and the hot water. Indeed, taking cold showers in the morning can be traced back to good old Kneipp, who believed them to be extremely beneficial. Thanks, Sebastian.

If you visit a spa where there are jacuzzis, plunge pools, cold water paddling, cool pools and hot pools alongside each other, or basins to place one arm in cold and the other in hot, then it is following Kneipp's ideas. Kneipp believed that hydrotherapy and thermotherapy are essentials for healthy bodies. There is a centre in Bad Wörishofen in Germany where you can study his work and experience his amazing and invigorating treatments.

You can try your own Kneipp treatments at home. They are very simple and hugely effective.

Bowl bathing

Take two large bowls – washing-up bowls will do. Fill one with ice-cold water and one with bath-temperature hot water – hot but not too hot.

Either put on your bathrobe or roll up your trousers.

Place both feet in the hot water for 2 minutes. Then immediately place both feet in the cold water for 2 minutes. Repeat this 5 times so that you are in both hot and cold for a total of 10 minutes.

Then dry your feet and either get dressed or put your socks on.

See how invigorated and relaxed you feel, both at the same time? The combination of hot and cold is totally balancing. Kneipp at home – well done.

In the bath

Run a hot bath, as hot as you are comfortable in. Turn the shower to a cold setting. Place an absorbent bathmat on the floor of your bathroom between the two. Undress. Get into the hot bath for 3 minutes. Get out without drying yourself and immediately get into the shower for 1 minute. Get straight back into the bath for 2 minutes, and then back in the shower for 1 minute. Repeat 5 times so that you have bathed Kneipp style. No trips to Germany, no foreign exchange, just the most revitalising bath you can ever experience – a true tonic.

Sauna and Steam

Water doesn't just come in flow form. In the introduction to this book I showed that water is so versatile, that there are millions of ways in which we can experience it. It's not just something we drink or wash in, or wash things with. Drinking and washing are only the tip of the iceberg (which is also water).

Another way of using water to detox is sauna and steam. Sauna and steam help you sweat out the toxins from within and cleanse your skin at the same time, the former with dry heat and the latter with wet heat. Saunas and steamrooms are widely available. Hotels and gyms are almost guaranteed to have at least one to enjoy, if not both. The use of heat is greatly beneficial and very relaxing indeed. If you can combine it with either a cold shower or plunge pool then your treatment is even more therapeutic and a little more enlivening, to say the least. As we're beginning to see, the combination of hot and cold is very healing internally and emotionally.

In a sauna, stones or rocks are heated so much that when water is poured over them they generate a dry, drawing heat. In a steamroom, water is heated so much that it begins to evaporate – just like the steam from a kettle can be pumped into an enclosed room and create a wet heat.

Both types of heat are designed to cleanse. The steamroom and sauna will cause the body to sweat. This will draw toxins out through the pores of the skin and cleanse any waste or build-up of oils and so on within the skin pores – which is especially good if you have blocked pores or skin prone to spots.

You can accelerate the effectiveness of a sauna or steam by using your favourite essential oils, essences or other natural products (see page 96–7 for recommended detox oils and herbs). You inhale and absorb much more effectively when your body is relaxed and warm.

The heating of the body causes vasodilation – the blood vessels relax and open wide, enabling blood to flow freely around the body (see page 79–80). If you use essential oils, their effect becomes deeper because of the enhanced circulation. You can just rub them into the surface of the skin: the blend will nourish the outer layers while the molecules of the essential oils will be inhaled or absorbed deep into the brain or bloodstream to take effect.

What we have to remember is that it is the short-term effects of the heat that we can benefit most from. You should spend no more than 15 minutes, on average, in a sauna or steamroom, and then you should either cool down naturally or, to get the best effect, jump into a plunge pool or take an ice-cold shower. Alternating the temperatures will increase and enhance the body's ability to heal itself immensely.

Take yourself off to the local gym or swimming pool and indulge in a sauna and steam session.

Jacuzzi

In a jacuzzi, heated water bubbles away in a tub or tank with jets of water aimed at specific points on the body to aid in massage and circulation. The water is usually quite warm, so you experience every aspect of heat application, and it is moving or being pushed out in jets that can actually massage the body or specific muscle and help it to relax if you sit against them. Again, the whole experience can be maximised if an oil, herbal remedy or tincture is added to the water. This will encourage full absorbency and therefore full benefit of the chosen product.

Alternating the hot jacuzzi with sessions in a plunge pool, cold shower, snowbank, or any other cold-water application will give the best results.

At this point it has to be said that cold showers, cold plunge pools and so on have had a bad press, and smack of health torture. But this is a false picture. While nearly every one of us has experienced the comforting and nurturing feelings that come with the application of heat, even if just from a relaxing warm shower, not many of us have taken the treatment to its full efficacy and added cold. Not many of us have actually been brave enough to partner the heat with the cool – the refreshing cold shower, jumping in the daunting plunge pool, pulling the string to empty the contents of the ice-cold water bucket over our bodies, or simply turning the shower to cool after washing in a hot shower. This will increase the results beyond belief.

Warm, in other words, is only half the story. I admit, warm is soooo nice; everything that warm does is comforting and relaxing, and it just makes us feel good inside. So, warm up, have lots of heat – and then add a little cold. Then warm up some more, then just a little cold. Warm up one last time and finish with a blast of cold, and I can guarantee you that the buzz your body will get from the alternate temperature will have your systems firing on all cylinders and your circulation so invigorated that you will feel warm all over for days to come.

The real beauty of it is, if you do it often enough, you will naturally improve your circulation, which will mean that you will feel a lot warmer most of the time. Think of the money you will save on heating bills!

Now for a look at treatments that concentrate less on temperature than on reaching the parts others can't.

Colonic Irrigation

Although it's been around since 1500 B.C., colonic irrigation seems to be a relatively new and experimental therapy to most people.

Colonic irrigation is an internal bath that helps to cleanse the colon of accumulated poisons, gases, faecal matter and mucus deposits. The practitioner will gently pump filtered water into the rectum, and this will start to soften and flush away any unwanted build-up of toxins and waste.

It is an extremely effective addition to any detox programme. During the programme you eliminate any source of toxins from your diet; this means that all toxins are being processed and eliminated, and not being replaced. Foodstuffs such as brown rice, nuts and pulses all help to break the built-up toxins down, and colonic irrigation will speed up this process by actively flushing out any matter.

The colonics practitioner will ask you to lie on a couch or plinth, with your lower body covered with a towel or sheet. Filtered water at a carefully regulated temperature is introduced under gentle gravitational pressure through the rectum and into the colon. The practitioner will use massage to help the water soften and cleanse the colon of faecal matter and waste that is flushed away with the waste water.

The colon is worked on in stages. Each time water is pumped in and flushed out until the whole area is complete. The treatment will last less than an hour and the modesty of the client is observed throughout the treatment: practitioners are totally aware of the 'unusual' circumstances of the procedure. It is then usual for the practitioner to recommend how many further treatments are required, and also which supplements to use to replace natural bowel fibre and flora.

The after-effects of colonic irrigation are similar to those of the entire Water Detox programme: a feeling of wellbeing, lightness, mental clarity, increased energy, loss of any bloated feeling, relief from constipation and clearer, glowing skin.

Colonics is not something that normally springs to mind as a complementary therapy – we usually think of massage or aromatherapy – but if you have ever thought about trying this treatment to see what the effects would be, or if you believe that this would help but have never got around to booking a session, then this is the time to try! It's painless, it's different, it makes you feel great, and it is detoxifying.

Walking by the Sea

Go to the seaside, walk by the shore or simply look at the crashing waves. Breathe in the air. Expand your horizons. Watch the tide ebb and flow and see how this reflects our lives – everything in balance.

The call of the sea is very common. You don't have to be a mariner to wish to go to the seaside to walk and refresh yourself. Now we hardly ever mean actually bathing in the sea; we seem to be able to benefit from it just by being by it or looking at it. We now know that this is because we can benefit from the vibration and resonance: the energy of the sea quite simply gets to us. Many hundreds of people buy a holiday home near the sea, or retire to the coast, or just visit the sea on a regular basis to share its immense energy.

Anyone who works on the sea will tell you of the huge respect you need to have for it. Its tides are controlled by the sun and moon, but apart from this it is a law unto itself. It can change from a millpond to a raging, crashing brute in just hours, and it can take lives in moments if the right care is not taken.

Anyone who thinks they are in charge of this deep, mysterious being can think again. Maybe this is the secret of its therapeutic effect. Maybe the gentle ripple or the strong crashing of the waves is what makes us feel mortal and humble again. The sea is a product of Mother Nature and we can only look on in wonder. It has its own life force, it gives life to an entire underwater world that operates by its own laws, and it has inspired much of the world's mythology. People even choose to be buried at sea. It is one of the strongest elements and it keeps us guessing. We can share some of that strength and power just by spending time at the seaside.

Watsu

Watsu is a form of water bodywork partly based on Zen Shiatsu, and created 20 years ago by Harold Dull. The treatments are quite amazing, even magical in effect. Watsu incorporates the use of water to support the body while a practitioner takes you through a balletic sequence of moves and stretches. It combines the experience of being in a flotation tank with gentle exercise and stretches, and is very sensuous. You are aware of the noises around you and the movement of the water near your ears. You are aware of your body being moved into different positions and gently gliding from one move to another as a stretch is held, then released. The whole experience lies somewhere between flying and floating. Truly wonderful and less passive than flotation.

Watsu treatments will help improve flexibility and are great for stretching muscles without the pressure of body weight. The real beauty of the Watsu treatment, however, is its ability to return your own body to the state of being inside your mother's womb. It is at once nurturing and releasing. The water is at a similar temperature to that of a flotation tank, so you lose all sense of being in the water: you feel suspended but you are not aware of what is keeping you floating or flying. The water ripples against your ears as you are moved and cradled but it never splashes your face; this means that the sound is underneath the water not above. Your hearing is dampened by the water, any noise is far away, and the only sound you are truly conscious of is the water in your head and the water in your ears. It is an experience I fully recommend, and certainly every pregnant woman should experience Watsu as it must give the truest indication of how their growing baby feels inside their womb.

Swimming with Dolphins

It's remarkable to experience the creatures of the deep at close hand, and connect to nature through the power of water. You hear the resonance of their sound waves and the vibrations of their bodies moving near you and around you. Many people talk of the wonder of swimming with dolphins or going on a voyage to see whales swimming in their natural habitat. And there is something mystical about these intelligent animals. When people have swum with these beautiful creatures, they often say it has quite fundamentally changed their lives.

What a fabulous way to stay young. To reassess your own life and to put things into perspective. To recapture your own youth. To be able to resonate and vibrate with these healing creatures must be unbelievable and incredibly emotional.

The actual experience of even seeing live dolphins is quite amazing. I have only seen dolphins swimming alongside a boat when I was on holiday with a big group of friends in Turkey. It was 6 o'clock in the morning and the crew was shouting and whooping about them. I got up and stumbled onto the deck to be totally mesmerised by the sheer beauty, speed and grace of them. You couldn't actually see how they were moving along so fast in front of the bow of the boat. Nothing was wobbling, nothing flapping and no fins moving that you could see. Their sheer power and grace was able to propel them with what seemed like no effort whatsoever.

All I do know was that in the time I was watching them, nothing else featured. I was in a place that was occupied only by the dolphins and me. No worries about anything, just the thrill of watching the amazing qualities of nature and appreciating its beauty.

It was fabulous fun, it made me want to giggle like a child, and it was very exciting – which for me, at 6 a.m., is pretty incredible in itself, I can assure you.

If you get the chance to make the booking during your 18 days, do so. If you don't, then just put the idea in your memory file and if you ever get the chance, grab it. There is a contact number at the back of this book to ensure that your experience is just as good for the dolphins as it is for you.

Bathing with a Difference

Introduce bathing into your life and actually think about it and how it feels. Here are three ways in which you can totally detox and transform yourself simply by taking a bath.

Candle bathing

You have probably done this already. The popularity of candlelight and the relaxation of a warm bath combined with a little peace and quiet is one of the easiest ways to experience hydrotherapy at home.

You have probably experienced it without truly understanding what it is doing for you.

The warm water is calmer than cool water, the candlelight is easier on the eye than a bulb, and the closed door prevents any interruption or outside disruption.

If you add essential oils to the water, you'll have the most relaxing experience in just a few moments. You'll find some ideas for which essential oils to use on page 86.

You can add to the total experience by scattering flower petals on the water – rose petals are just beautiful for this. As the warm water surrounds the flowers, the fragrance mixes with the steam and can be easily inhaled.

Using Bach Rescue Remedy or other floral essences can enhance the water's vibration and so the benefit to you. Crystal elixirs will have a similar effect – relaxing or calming. Whatever you wish for, choose the essence and drop it into your bath.

Run a bath that is hot enough to stay warm for 15 to 20 minutes, but not so hot it is uncomfortable to sit in.

When your bath is full, let the water become still, then sprinkle a tablespoon of blended oil, essential oil, flower essence, crystal spritz or flower petals, or a combination of all of them, over the water.

Close all the windows so that none of the steam escapes, then light your candles to create a really relaxing, sensuous experience. Slowly get into the bath and once in, concentrate on breathing slowly and deeply, inhaling all the vapours. Allow your skin to soak and absorb all the resonance and vibration. You should be able to totally relax and unwind. Try to detox your mind at this time as well as your body. If thoughts enter, then simply let them exit!

Once you have finished the bath, get out slowly. Pat yourself dry, allowing as much of the moisture as you can to stay on your flesh, acting as a natural moisturiser and allowing any residual oil to continue to be absorbed. If you need to dress after you bathe, you should moisturise to help keep in the residual moisture. Ideally you should now relax or go straight to bed! Warm water is calming, so don't attempt any fast moves.

Revitalising Refresher

Run your bath in exactly the same way as described above. You do not need to light the candles, but you should play some invigorating and upbeat music directly outside the bathroom – but do not take an electrical unit into the bathroom.

Have ready the following ingredients:
Half a lemon for squeezing
3 drops lemon essential oil
2 drops peppermint essential oil
3 drops pine essential oil
Half a lemon, cut into thin slices
1 peppermint teabag

Squeeze the juice of the half-lemon into a teaspoon and mix in the essential oils. Sprinkle this mixture into the water. Scatter the lemon slices on the water and drop in the peppermint teabag. Wait 2 minutes for your bath to 'brew', then squeeze the teabag out into the water. Discard the used bag.

Get into the bath and breathe deep, slow breaths. Feel your body come alive and feel refreshed and invigorated. It's like immersing in a vat of your very own Water Detox tea!

When you get out of the bath, you should be ready for just about anything and smell pretty good too!

Ginger Warmer

This bath was described to me as an all-round tonic. If you have had a hard day or if the Water Detox programme has uncovered a little too much 'tox', then this is the bath for you.

Take one large piece of fresh ginger root. You can buy these in most supermarkets. Grate the root into a pulp or cut into lots of very thin slices. Leave yourself 2 or 3 slices and put to one side. Run your bath so that it is quite hot but bearable for you to sit in.

Mix the grated or sliced ginger into the water. Close the windows and doors so that the ginger infusion can get into the air. While this is happening, take the remaining ginger and mix into a mug of hot water. Go back to the bathroom, get into the bath and sip your ginger tea while lazing in the bath.

When you get out of the bath you should go to bed or wrap up warm and sit for an hour. This bath is fabulous for purging toxins, improving digestion and expelling bad germs, aches and pains.

Try to take at least one of these baths each week and see just how different they can make you feel.

Invigorating Showers

A swim in a cool pool, sea or lake every morning would be ideal for the Water Detox. But we can get similar results from a cool shower. Shower water is the exact opposite of bath water. It is fast-flowing and invigorating. I have always supported the idea of starting the day with a cold shower and now I know so much more about just why, I can continue to go on about this subject. There is no doubt that it lends us tremendous vigour – physical, mental, emotional and spiritual.

The cold water will increase your circulation, tone muscles and skin, and give the lymph a jumpstart. We've seen how cold water is much more energising than hot water. The molecules are much more excited in fast-flowing water than they are in slow-moving or still water. We will pick up on this resonance and vibration. There is a reason why we shower in the morning to wake up, and relax in a hot bath to soothe and calm. We just didn't know what it was!

If you have ever taken a shower or bath somewhere where there was no hot water, you will remember that it actually left you considerably warmer than it would have done if you had taken a normal hot shower. Indeed, in hot weather it is more effective to take a shower that is lukewarm or blood temperature rather than cold, as a cold shower will increase your circulation and warm you up, not cool you down.

If you happen to live by the sea, any chance you get you should take off your shoes and paddle – but just for 2 minutes tops. We don't want any reports of frostbite!

If you choose invigorating showers for your hydrotherapy experience, here are a few suggestions for kick-starting the day.

The Invigorator

Get into a hot shower and wash as normal. Using a soap or body exfoliator of your choice, wash quite vigorously to stimulate the skin. Once the washing is over, turn the shower to cold. Do not move out of the water but stand for a count of 10. Then turn the tap back to hot as it was before. Count to 5. Turn back to cold and stand for the count of 10 again.

Turn the shower off and get out. Rub your body vigorously with the towel and dress as normal.

You will soon feel invigorated, awake, alive and very, very warm. Your circulation, lymph and skin have been given a total workout – well done!

The Moisturiser

Warm up your bathroom so that it is comfortable to sit in while you're naked. Grate the zest of a whole lime and mix together with 2 large tablespoons of honey and the juice of the lime. Take this blend and smooth it all over your body as a wonderfully nourishing and moisturising body polish.

Sit for at least 5 minutes and preferably 10, but don't get cold. If you are prepared to wash your robe then you could put this on for extra warmth if your bathroom isn't up to full heat. (Ideally do this if you have access to a sauna or steamroom.)

Once the time is up, get into a warm shower and wash away the mix. Emerge moisturised and glowing.

Remember: you only need to choose three hydrotherapy treatments as part of your Water Detox. You will feel the toxins wash away.

OILS AND HERBS FOR THE WATER DETOX PROGRAMME

Essential oils

Neroli	Uplifting and stimulating.
Lavender	Relaxing and sleep inducing. Relieves stress and calms a troubled mind.
Sandalwood	Antidepressant, uplifting and very positive.
Grapefruit	Fruity and refreshing; a very positive oil.
Eucalyptus	Kills germs, wards off illness, and is balancing and energising.
Rosemary	Very balancing and grounding.

Herbs

If you wish to use the essential oils of these herbs, you can do so in place of the actual fresh leaves.

Fennel   Diuretic and balancing; tasty too.

Parsley   Cleansing, antioxidant and refreshing.

Coriander   A digestive that will help with cleansing the gut.

Sage   Extremely strong and very purging and cleansing; especially contraindicated in pregnancy.

Tarragon   Relaxing and calming, this herb will also help cleanse your digestive system.

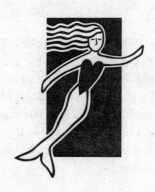

4

Thalassotherapy

THE WORD *THALASSA* IS THE Greek for 'sea', and thalassotherapy is the name given specifically to treatments involving seawater and minerals. During the 18-day Water Detox, we recommend that you try 3 types of thalassotherapy. You should spread them out across the 18 days and plan them alongside the other treatments you should be doing. You can go for professional treatments, or you can do them for yourself at home.

- Seaweed wraps
- Seawater bathing
- Spa thalassotherapy
- Cold algae
- Sea salt exfoliation
- Clay or mud treatments
- Flotation
- Dead sea bathing

First, you should see just how nutritious thalassotherapy can be for your body. We are 75 per cent water, and our bodies and minds are likely to be affected in exactly the same way as the moon affects the tides, as we are emotionally and physically affected by the gravitational changes. We have seen also that water can be affected by the vibrations and resonance of almost anything that we mix with it, place by it, or submerge in it.

If the content of the water is already rich in minerals, vibrations and resonance we do not need to do anything to it to get great benefits from it. We cannot fail to be wonderfully nourished and balanced ourselves if we use this highly nutritious water in our everyday life.

Seawater is just such water. The minerals in it are highly nutritious and extremely therapeutic.

You can practise thalassotherapy at home, in a spa, or even just by using a product that you introduce into your normal skin or body care routine. However you find them, they should be in your life.

Thalassotherapy combines every beneficial aspect of hydrotherapy, and adds the rich minerals and salts of the sea. Thalassotherapy takes hydrotherapy to the next stage. The optimum thalassotherapy treatments are those given with what is known as 'live' or 'fresh' seawater, which is directly pumped from the sea itself to, say, a spa.

It's the mineral content that is seawater's magic ingredient. The constituents of seawater are said to be similar to those of blood plasma, so spending time immersed or absorbing these minerals and salts is extremely beneficial for our health. Blood plasma is the fluid in our bodies that feeds and nourishes our cells, and helps health and wellbeing.

Many of the nutrients in seawater perform different and combined functions in the body: iron, zinc, calcium, magnesium, sodium, potassium, sulphur, selenium, nickel, iodine and aluminium. These minerals can balance the body's metabolism and thyroid function, relax and relieve muscle fibre, help enormously with cellulite, boost circulation, reduce stress and totally relax (see the table on page 100–102). The Dead Sea is one of the most popular healing destinations for this very reason: it contains enormous amounts of minerals and salts. If you simply float in these waters you will absorb the goodness and emerge feeling renewed and rejuvenated.

Thalassotherapy doesn't just concern seawater. It uses all the constituents of the sea, such as seaweed, which is extremely rich in iodine, pure and invigorating sea air, sea clay, mud and sea salt. Used to its full potential, thalassotherapy is a cure-all.

The buoyant quality of salt-rich seawater is an added bonus. The Dead Sea's famous buoyancy allows swimmers to float as if weightless when in the water. This is ideal if you wish to alleviate, regenerate, or manipulate damaged or injured muscles. The same qualities can be found in salt or brine baths. These are often used for remedial or physiotherapeutic treatments, as they take the weight and strain off the muscles and aid in freer movement.

You can even drink the stuff. There is nothing new in 'taking the waters' – a phrase that originated in the 18th century, but is a concept harking back to ancient Rome. Spa towns have always combined the benefits of freshwater and saltwater treatments to facilitate all-round healing. The seawater goes through some levels of purification in order to be palatable, but the rich mineral content – especially that of selenium, which is a potent antioxidant – makes taking the waters a topical and relevant treatment in itself.

Thalassotherapy treatments don't always use cold seawater. They are used at varying temperatures to enable the body to absorb the minerals more efficiently. If you combine the endless benefits of thalassotherapy with the principles of thermotherapy, you can begin to see that spa treatments are essential to maintaining a balanced and healthy body – and quite nice too! What a fabulous excuse to book yourself in.

Let's take a closer look at the minerals and what they do.

Minerals in seawater	Function
Bromides	Cell regeneration, repair and metabolism. Build immunity and recovery after injury.
Calcium	Regulates the heart and the nervous system. Nourishes bones and teeth. Especially helps arthritis sufferers and the elderly. It works with magnesium to keep muscles and nerves

functioning efficiently and helps the body regulate pH balance (alkalinity/acidity).

Iodine, Nickel, Aluminium

Their main function is balance and regulation. Balanced thyroid function keeps the body's hormone production balanced and a balanced metabolism acts as a natural antiseptic to aid skin conditions.

Magnesium

Magnesium strengthens bones and teeth, and promotes muscle health and therefore heart health. Magnesium is needed for the correct metabolism of sodium and potassium. Optimum function of these two minerals is essential. Magnesium is required for all cell activity and is also great for drawing toxins out of the body. It also helps the metabolism of calcium and if it is deficient then calcium deposits occur, as kidney stones, for instance.

Potassium

Combined with sodium, this mineral maintains fluid balance within the body. Potassium expels excess fluids and also plays an important role in cell metabolism, nerve and muscle responses, and general muscle health and hydration.

Selenium

An extremely potent antioxidant. Often combined with vitamins A, C, and E, selenium is top choice for protecting your body against free radicals, thus boosting total immunity. It protects against carcinogens and promotes heart health.

Sodium

Partnered with potassium, this mineral acts as a pump to maintain fluid levels within the body. Sodium absorbs and potassium expels, essential for maintaining blood pressure and even reputed to combat cellulite and water retention. It is essential that the balance between potassium and sodium be maintained to create the optimum 'pump' of fluids in the body.

Sulphur	Known mostly for its unpleasant smell, sulphur aids liver metabolism and detoxification. It also helps in the formation of blood vessels, tones the skin, keeps hair and nails healthy, and helps the body fight bacterial infection.
Zinc	Zinc is essential for health, promoting healing, growth, a healthy nervous system, development of bones and teeth and all-round energy levels.

Now for a perusal of the treatments and what they can do.

Thalassotherapy treatment	Benefits
Algotherapy, seaweed wraps	Wrapping the body in products containing marine algae aids the circulation and cleansing internally and externally.
	You can apply these treatments at home by purchasing seaweed powders and mixing them with water to a paste. However, these can be messy and are perhaps better as a professional treatment. So book yourself in now for a seaweed treatment.
Baths	Relaxing bathing in seawater to absorb minerals and nutrients that feed the body and balance fluid and metabolism.
	To DIY sea bathe, try an Epsom salts bath. Remember, wrap up warm after the treatment and feel the toxins creep out of every pore.
Balneotherapy	Heated bathing including the use of water jets and moving water – a seawater jacuzzi, if you like.

Difficult to do at home, so try to save this for a professional spa visit.

Brumisation

Treatments incorporating inhalation of sea mist to benefit from internal invigoration and cleansing.

Again, not something that can be done easily at home.

Cryotherapy

Application of cold algae products to the body in a wrap reduces water retention by expelling excess fluids, and boosts circulation. Most popular for immediate reduction in body measurements and treating cellulite.

There are many professional product ranges that can be taken at day spas and salons. There are also many products available from body care shops and chemists that can be applied to more accessible parts of the body – thighs, hips, arms and so on. Not too messy, but better in small areas.

Body/exfoliating scrubs

Sea salts mixed with essential oils, base oils or other complementary sea/algae products, designed to smooth and soften the skin and increase circulation. They slough away dead skin cells to encourage glowing skin.

Home use is easy. There are hundreds of exfoliation products containing salts and oils. Alternatively, you can mix natural sea salts in flake or granular form together with an oil or cream to make your own DIY version. I have included exfoliation recipes on pages 127–128.

Wraps, clay and deep-sea mud	Drawing and cleansing. Using sea mud or clay, these treatments are extremely high in the same minerals as the sea, but the substance and texture of the mud and clay is good for painting onto the body or using as a treatment wrap to cleanse and detox.
	Again, you can buy products from your local chemists' or beauty departments, and application in localised areas is easier than attempting to try to do your whole body.
Flotation	Book into your local float centre and drift away.
Dead sea bathing	Go on: treat yourself, pick up a brochure next time you're out. You deserve it.

Salt bathing and flotation tanks are not traditionally considered as pure thalassotherapy. This is because they do not use natural seawater or sea products. I have included them in this section, however, because of their concentrated use of minerals and salts. Bathing uses natural salts added to water, and flotation uses huge concentrations of salts for their buoyancy purposes.

SALT BATHING

Also known as cleansing salts, magnesium bathing and Epsom salts, this is a way of purging your body of toxins by simply bathing in salt-water.

There are ways to use salt bathing at home. Epsom salts baths are just as effective as many seawater baths.

Epsom salts are pure magnesium, and this mineral is an essential requirement for nearly all of our cellular activity. Bathing in Epsom salts allows the skin to absorb the magnesium. The magnesium will also absorb or 'draw' toxins from the body, so it is likely that you will 'glow' with perspiration for a while after your bath. This will not be quite a sweat – unless you wrap up really warm! It is more likely that you'll feel as if you are in a very humid room. It is very important to keep warm, not only to increase the effect of the magnesium, but also to prevent you from catching a chill. Epsom salts baths will improve circulation, too.

The Epsom salts bath can be extremely relaxing and warming, helping to soothe aching joints and muscles. Taken before bed, this will almost certainly guarantee the deepest night's sleep!

FLOTATION

Flotation is a fabulous relaxation tool. The high salt content of the flotation water is similar to that of the sea. Mineral and sea salts make the water used very buoyant and enable us to float.

One of the ultimate water experiences we have all had, without any doubt whatsoever, is being inside the womb. Everyone has spent time in the womb, in the amniotic sac of fluid, suspended and floating.

A successful flotation session is often described as returning to the womb. The similarities are there: the sensation of warmth in your mother's womb from floating in blood-temperature water, suspended in fluids, with no sound except the heartbeat of your mother. The only guaranteed sense or sound in a flotation experience will be your own heart beating and other noises emanating from your own body.

Flotation is a brilliant way of having your cares washed away, and returning to basics and what really matters. Flotation takes everything away from you, including smell, vision, sound, body awareness and weight, and then just gives you a clear space in your head to either concentrate on one thing or truly clear your mind – to totally float away.

Whatever you read about flotation, it still seems hard to believe that you will truly feel totally weightless and stressless, as the marketing material insists. Well, try it just once and you will immediately, or very soon, see that it works. It is very similar to meditation. You need to clear your mind of everything and anything – to let your mind, body and spirit clear. But with meditation, you need to be in a warm room, with no disturbances – children, partners, phone, and so on – and you need to sit or lie in one place for a reasonable period of time. There lies the rub: as humans, we are not designed to stay still for any period of time at all. We are designed to move and respond and react, so for a lot of people meditation is very difficult for periods longer than 10 minutes, even though you need longer to focus effectively.

The beauty of flotation is that you are suspended in water, so the aches and pains and actual stress of mobility are taken away. (Indeed, people who are normally not able-bodied can become totally free and flexible, and their once immoveable joints can just float and feel released. Small aches and pains feel like they are melting away, and large pains caused by weight bearing are released or greatly relieved.)

Flotation is also extremely relaxing as it takes away 90 per cent of our normal, continual stimulus. We look all the time, we move continually, we react to every little thing going on around us, we hear words and sounds that our minds think about, and we touch things and articles that register in our brains. We interact continually with our surroundings and even when we are doing one thing, we are probably thinking about another or about how to do something completely different. Because floatation takes every sense away, nothing is left except your own mind. Blood pressure is lowered and the heart rate slows down to a healthy pace.

So, floating, relaxed and with no stimulus and so nothing to respond to, the brain starts to relax and recuperate. And when it does it naturally begins to balance out. Left-side brain function – the side that works out problems and logistics – relaxes and balances out with the underused right-side creative brain function. That is why the flotation technique is very popular with creative artists in search of inspiration and new ideas.

Even this activity becomes involuntary, which means the relaxation and balancing happens with no need for activity from ourselves. We just concentrate on nothing and let our bodies adjust, renew and regenerate. If we have no thoughts to process then we can truly, truly relax. The regeneration that comes with flotation is at once spiritual, emotional, mental and physical, and is a wonderful way of meditating.

The flotation experience has moved on in leaps and bounds from the once common plastic or glass fibre 'pod', which could be described as claustrophobic or simply dingy, and certainly not very 'natural'. I once heard it described as getting into a Robin Reliant parked down a wet, dark lane with the engine switched off! Definitely not the holistic, relaxing experience it could be.

Now, when you practise flotation you are more likely to enter a specially built room with tiles and steps in and out, with plenty of space for moving around and preparation. The room means you don't have to climb into anything dark and shut a lid, which a lot of people can find difficult – it does feel a bit like getting into a gloomy box. In today's flotation set-up, the room is generally very subtly lit and the lights fade down to off in the first few moments of your session. You can opt for them to be left on to make you feel safer if necessary, but there is a real feeling of nurturing when you float, so I am sure you will be happy to turn the lights off completely. There is also the option to have music or sound tapes playing during your float. Again, this is a matter of choice: you will probably choose to have something in the first few minutes but then try fading it out with the lighting so you can truly experience absolute peace.

Inside the tanks or rooms, the water is heated to blood temperature. This is important, as it means that after a short period of time you will no longer be able to feel the water. There is no difference between your body temperature and the water temperature – you will blend into your surroundings and probably won't even feel the water moving over the sides of your body.

The water is full of Epsom salts for buoyancy and softness. One concern of some people is that the flotation tank is a deep pool. In fact, a flotation pool is generally only 25 to 50 centimetres deep. There is absolutely no need for depth, as you are truly 'floating' on the surface.

Sports therapists benefit greatly from flotation, as it makes the muscles and limbs weightless and this helps the body to speed up the mending and rebuilding process. Brine baths are also used for physio-therapy, sports injuries and even equine injuries. Taking the weight away gives more range of movement or even just a first opportunity for movement.

And finally, as well as being totally relaxing and regenerating, flotation is extremely detoxing. Epsom salts bathing has long been recommended as one of the strongest cleansing and drawing techniques we can use on our bodies.

Below is your thalassotherapy treatment checklist. Remember to choose 3 for Water Detox.

- Seaweed wraps
- Spa therapies
- Cold algae
- Sea salt/exfoliation
- Clay or mud treatment
- Flotation
- Sea bathing – real or 'at home Epsom salts'

5

Watercise

I MAKE NO BONES ABOUT the fact that I am not particularly keen on exercise. I love the benefits, the toned body, the feeling of fitness, and the thought that I am keeping my body healthy. I love the feeling just after a workout because I know it is over until the next time. I love the company of the people I exercise with. I just can't seem to like the exercise.

If I look at it in a different way, making the exercise into an activity, then I can think about it quite differently. I like gardening: that gets my body working; I like decorating: the times I go up and down the ladder must count for something; I love taking city breaks and walking for days just looking around. None of this is exercise as such, but it is all most definitely healthy activity for the body. If we combine the idea of exercise as just another activity, with water, then we can see that there are many possibilities for getting fit and healthy.

Over the next 18 days you should look to include some form of water activity every other day. That's 9 days of activity in total.

Being able to swim opens up a world of opportunities for recreation on the water. There's sailing, windsurfing, water-skiing, speed boating, flotilla holidays, canoeing, white-water rafting, and more that I haven't even heard of. To feel comfortable in water is to be able to open up a whole new world of ways to get fit and become active without actually exercising for exercise's sake.

Most water sports are open to people who don't swim as the safety precautions taken mean that there is no opportunity for anything to go wrong: even swimmers are required to wear life-saving jackets and waistcoats, for instance. However, the knowledge that you are comfortable in the water means you are more likely to enjoy the experience rather than be apprehensive about it.

Getting into the swim is imperative to the Water Detox. It cleanses inside and outside and it gets us very much in the flow and in touch with how our bodies feel, with none of the physical or mental stresses that we put on our bodies every day.

GETTING ON TO AND INTO THE WATER

Contact numbers for most of these categories are listed at the back of the book (see page 198).

Swimming

Swimming should make us feel wonderfully natural and free. It combines activity with the vibration of water and the support of the fluids carrying our bodies effortlessly along.

We do not actually swim in the womb, but we are suspended in fluid. We cannot swim naturally once we are born but the sooner we get into the water and start to learn to swim the more easily we do become natural swimmers. There can be a huge fear of water if we have not learnt how to swim from an early age. In order to swim, to physically let go of a handrail or hand, we need to trust that we can float. We trust implicitly when we are born, but we learn to mistrust each time something goes against our natural belief. If we fail to learn to swim until we are adult, then we have learnt to fear and not to trust the beauty of water.

If you are a parent, give your child the beauty of swimming as soon as you can. Call your local pool and get the sessions sorted now. If you are not so young or just want to learn to swim, do the same – adult swimming lessons are just as numerous as children's in most pools and you will be able to share the experience with people at the same level of competence.

There really is no excuse not to be able to swim. Fear of the water can easily be overcome if you take the steps to learn slowly and safely, and the enjoyment and freedom of swimming will far outweigh any self-doubt you may have. If you can conquer this one, then you really can do anything you want to in this world. So get in the swim.

Swimming is definitely not *just* swimming. Swimming tones the body from top to toe. The muscles in the arms become stronger and more streamlined as they pull your body through the water. Your hips and thighs are worked in every stroke and the muscles become leaner. Swimming can strengthen the back as it is used to support the body in the water. Upper and lower body strength is developed in swimming, as well as aerobic capacity. Swimming works the entire body but without the pounding and pressure of 'land-based' exercise.

Once you have gained confidence in the water, you have opened up a fabulous new world of opportunities. You can relax, take exercise, increase lymph flow, increase the range of muscle work, and exercise in a weight-free environment to help with injury.

The sky (or the sea) is the limit: swimming for relaxation, meditation, exercise or sport, paddling in the pool with your children, water fights, water polo, aqua aerobics, synchronised swimming, diving, snorkelling and probably many, many more.

Contact your local leisure centre for information on how you can get in the swim. Choose your watery activity and savour the experience.

Sailing

Sailing can be both exhilarating and relaxing. The vibration of racing water is so different from that of the calm millpond of the bay, but both are the sea. It is the vibration that causes the different effects of relaxation or exhilaration. Sailing in a race will use the surface of the water and the wind to generate speed and flow, cutting through the ocean waves and pitting your skill against the elements. Feel the spray of the water tingling on your skin and splashing you into life, blowing the cobwebs away. On the other hand, sailing in a beautiful boat around some Mediterranean islands, stopping off in coves and bays to enjoy the tranquillity, will bring total relaxation and recuperation.

If you decide to take sailing as your watercise, you need to become involved in crewing. Under instruction you will soon find out that the rigorous demands on the body while handling the boat in even the slightest breeze will open up the lungs, tighten the leg muscles and strengthen the arms. There is nothing passive about crewing a sailboat. Adrenaline pumping through the veins and blood coursing around the body is an all-round workout.

If you decide that sailing at any level would be an interesting way to introduce watersports into your life contact the Royal Yachting Association (see page 198). Make sure your boat club is recognised and you will make sure your sailing is safe.

Canoeing

Canoeing is a remarkable option. Be tested by the water and the underlying current to win out against the fast-moving river, cutting into small areas, rolling over and righting to race down a small gap between treacherous rocks to be spewed out into a wide area of river to gently flow along until the next test is encountered. The water froths and chops and generates adrenaline and excitement, then, as it calms down, cools and calms the canoeist.

Canoeing develops upper-body strength and agility. Your waistline will be tested as you twist and turn along the route, and it will certainly work your back and arms. Anything to get the circulation pumping and increase the heart rate will benefit both mind and body.

Windsurfing

Take a board out on the water to harness the power of the wind in order to fly along. You'll find yourself going with and against the wind's flow. The windsurfer is alone on the water but reliant on it just the same. Water carries them along and lends exhilaration and speed. Then the wind drops and the windsurfer drops into the water, to be totally enveloped by the element that supports them.

If you have ever tried to windsurf, you will know that it uses every muscle in your body as well as truly testing your mind. Even muscles you didn't know you had will be worked. From picking up the sail to pulling yourself out of the water to getting onto the board, it's a challenge. When you are eventually in full sail, you will need all the strength you can muster to hold on as you cut through the waves at high speed.

Skiing

Snow, after all, is just water in a solid state. The snow carries the skier quickly along the surface, cutting through with the edge of the skis and sending a spray of snow up and out behind in a wake. The light and energy of the snow generates freshness and vitality.

Skiing is similar to windsurfing: every muscle in the lower and upper body is required at some time. Even the jaws get a good workout, as you shout with excitement racing down through the fresh powder snow and bouncing among the moguls. Legs, thighs, arms, stomach and heart, all get a thorough workout.

Diving

In a sense, diving is travelling to the unknown under the water. It's all about feeling the strength and the pressure of the water as you go deeper, feeling and hearing the silence and seeing the whole system and forms of life that survive without ever breathing a breath.

Terrifying and exciting at the same time, diving gives a true picture of another world – the fish and the coral, the geography, the reefs and the caves, the wrecks and the caverns. But diving isn't about water as a medium. It is rarely about the texture of the water and the fact that you are immersed in it. Water is the only reason we can dive, but when diving we don't think about it except for its potential danger.

Diving takes on the resonance of deep water, which puts you in contact with deep thoughts and awareness of other worlds. Experienced divers talk of deep calm and tranquillity and of the otherworldliness of the underwater world.

Diving is a more gentle form of exercise, but arms and legs will be toned and lengthened. You will glide through the water like a sleek fish and develop a slim body to match.

Waterfalls

Travelling long distances to see famous waterfalls, and including them in a trek, can be thought of as an unusual form of watercise. Think of Niagara and Victoria Falls. The power and the force of the water is at once terrifying and wonderful, exhilarating and energising. It is enough to pay hundreds of pounds to travel to the sight to have a picture taken or to even travel under the flow to get close to it. Let the water splash against your face or just look at the view and feel the force. It is both empowering and humbling – perhaps that is why we make the journey.

Walking Along a Riverbank, Stream or Brook

Taking a walk along the banks of a river or stream can give you entirely different experiences.

A river, with the water coursing slowly in mass, has a rhythm and flow of its own. It carries small boats and occupies fishermen and gives you the feeling of life from the water. People are drawn to the water and the steady, calming effect of that constant flow.

The busy babbling and chattering of a brook running through the fields, forests and woods, clean and fresh, light-hearted and with no major purpose, simply an overflow or a surge from the rainfall, is a wonderful contrast. Try to dam it, and it finds a way to escape and continue flowing every time. Somehow, the chattering and busyness of a brook invites you in to be industrious and light-hearted. No walk by the stream is right without ending in someone getting splashed or dunked or just a little too soggy.

The Swimming Pool

How about doing nothing except sitting by the pool with a good book? This doesn't sound much like exercise. But of course you can swim in it – and you can exercise your other faculties by it. You can look at the water and at its colour, you look at it move and you can smell it. It can cool you down, relax you, make you feel pampered or invite a whole new dimension of social interaction. If someone invites us round for the kids to play in the paddling pool, we accept. A water fight ensues but it is all about letting go, chilling out and enjoying water.

Moving in and with and by water can have a profound effect on us, there's no doubt. Pitting our strength against it, working with it, leaves us fitter and at the same time clearer-headed, calmer, more energised – and aesthetically satisfied. It's a win-win situation.

6

Youth Dew

BEAUTY IS AN ESSENTIAL COMPONENT of Water Detox: skin care and body care are big elements of the programme. Our skin, after all, is a reflection of how healthy we are. It is the biggest external organ, and it protects us. It is time we took care of it and nourished it with water.

Each day you will:

- Moisturise your entire body every morning.

- Dry skin brush your entire body every morning.

- Cleanse your face however you wish to, then splash it 3 times with warm water and 3 times with cold water.

- Spritz a mist of water over your skin before applying moisturiser every morning.

- Apply moisturiser twice a day and make sure it is at least 15 SPF.

You will also exfoliate your body and face every 3 days.

There are few secrets about looking good. Few, because we actually know exactly how to look good, but we still don't seem to find the time or motivation to do so!

- Eat a healthy diet rich in fruits, vegetables, grains and oily fish.

- If you smoke, stop.

- Moderate your alcohol intake.

- Protect your skin from UVA/UVB rays.

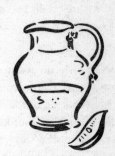

- Follow a skin care/body care programme.

- Exercise regularly.

- Hydrate.

WHAT'S IN THE SKIN

Typical human skin contains between 8 and 10 litres of water. The top layers of the skin contain 10 per cent of that, and the remainder is found in the lower layers. The fluid we drink travels to the lower layers, and if there is sufficient water in our bodies, the water is also able to reach the outer dermis – the bit that is on view. If we don't drink enough, supplies run out before it reaches our surface skin and we start to look dry and lines and wrinkles are much more accentuated. A glass of water an hour will ensure that these layers remain fully hydrated and plump, and lines simply melt away.

Our skin mirrors our body's internal state, so:

If we are tired	Our skin is pale
If we are stressed	Our skin is drained-looking
If we are unhappy	Our skin is dull
If we eat an unhealthy diet	We have spots and coloration around the chin
If we have hormonal imbalance	We have spots and breakouts

If we don't sleep	We get puffy eyes and pale faces
If we are healthy and happy	We have a rosy glow
If we are fit	We have toned and glowing skin
If we are totally hydrated	We have wrinkle-free, toned, plump, rosy, fresh and fabulous skin . . . Just 2 litres of water away . . .

Not only do we need to drink the water. We also need to keep the water we drink from escaping just as quickly as we drink it. We can help to keep our levels of hydration constant by regulating the amount of oil in the skin, known as sebum. If the oil is produced at the right rate, the skin stays normal, but if we overproduce oil then we get oily skin and obviously if we underproduce oil we get dry skin. This happens because the sebum acts as a barrier to water loss. If the barrier is insufficient, then of course water will escape. If the thin film of oil is balanced, the water stays in and the oil protects against any dryness. Remember, the surface area of the body is huge and water evaporates from this surface all day long. Covering up doesn't prevent the loss as we sweat fluids as well. The only answer to hydration is protection and fluid intake.

As soon as we apply a product to our face, we can disrupt the oil balance and thus disrupt the protective barrier. This is why most of the products we use on our faces contain some sort of oil or balancing substance to maintain this protection. We also need to be careful when cleansing. Stripping too much of the oil away will throw the skin's delicate balance into disarray. As the body tries to rectify the loss, it will rally to produce more oils, and then find that it is overcompensating because of an external factor.

In an ideal world, there would be no pollution and no make-up. We would eat healthily, the skin's natural oils would protect the epidermis and we would simply need to splash water on our faces to wash away the dust. However, we use make-up, we live in polluted air, even out in the countryside, and we are subjected to the sun's harmful rays. We need cleansers that will clean dirt and make-up without totally stripping the protective layers away.

The only way to find out exactly the right products for yourself is to have your skin analysed. Most skin care ranges will be able to offer this service free of charge. If they cannot then you should be concerned about their ability to sell you the right product.

MOISTURISING

Possibly the most important aspect of skin care is to keep the moisture levels right. This is done mainly from within – yes, by now it should be drilled into your heads that drinking a minimum of 2 litres of water a day will do the trick. But there is little point in feeding your body with water if you do not protect and moisturise your skin. It could be likened to pouring water into a jug with millions of minuscule holes in it. The job is never-ending. If you seal the skin with a fine film of oil, or even use a product that prevents moisture loss, you will be reducing the loss of up to 1 litre of water per day through your skin.

Partner this with sun protection and antioxidants, and you will be giving your skin a special treat every day of your life. You will also be making yourself look younger and more glowing into the bargain.

We have a huge choice of moisturisers and protection creams. The selection is totally mind-boggling, but there are a few that seem to have a specific and very useful purpose. After reading about them below, hopefully you will be able to settle on the right creams for you when you go for your skin analysis.

Alpha Hydroxy Acids (AHAs)

AHAs are fruit acids, lactic acids, glycolic acids – from sugar – and tartaric acids, from wine. All these acids are reputed to soften the skin and to increase its ability to hold moisture. Wine acids are becoming increasingly popular as research suggests that grape seeds and therefore any wine products are highly antioxidant and therefore rejuvenating or even able to reverse the signs of ageing.

Ceramides

The body naturally produces ceramides and certain types are found in the skin. Healthy skin has a good balance of ceramides but dry skin needs more. Applying them to the skin is intended to supplement the shortfall and thus improve the appearance and possibly the actual health of the skin. If they do not actually get absorbed into the skin they do seem to help protect and boost the skin's barrier.

Collagen

Collagen is commonly found in our make-up and cosmetics. It can hydrate the skin and it can also hold a fine layer of water on the skin's surface. It therefore serves as a valuable ingredient as it helps to improve the appearance of fine lines or simply boosts skin tone.

Humectants

Humectants can actually attract water from the atmosphere and hold it on the surface of the skin. This thin layer helps to prevent any loss of water from the skin's dermis.

Lipids

Lipids are fats. The fats in our skin's upper layers help to reduce water loss, so adding them to our skin care range can help to prevent loss of fluid. When we cleanse with extreme or stripping products and remove some of the essential fats from the protective layer on our skins, the lipids in our skin care products can help to replace the loss.

Retinoids and Retin A

Retinoids are vitamin A molecules. They are reported to actually increase the rate at which the body renews its skin cells. If there is sun or wind or any form of damage to the skin, using retinoids could just speed up the production of new skin cells and the discarding of old and damaged ones.

NATURAL PRODUCTS

There are ways to look after your skin quite naturally. You can use essential oils and skin care products made from natural ingredients. These can do everything the cosmetic versions can but without any of the manufactured chemicals.

Many of the natural nut, food or plant oils are very similar in make-up to the skin's natural sebum. Not too suprisingly, the foods that feed our skin from the outside are also all part of the 18-Day H_2O Nutrition Programme, except bananas. So put bananas on, but not in!

Taking these oils internally or applying them to the skin can help replace lost oils and encourage the body to produce more or less depending on what is required. The common myth is that you should not eat or add oils to oily skin, but if you add a natural oil such as jojoba or avocado, the body recognises the constituents and then begins to stop its own production. Natural oils are much more likely to regulate and balance the skin's own production of oil than manufactured products are. The nutrients supplied within are going to be much more effective than anything applied to the external surface. If you get the balance right then you can get your skin fully hydrated, nourished and protected.

Natural product	Benefits
Aloe vera	Softens skin, helps soothe sun damage.
Apricot kernel oil	Moisturises.
Avocado oil, avocado	Moisturises, supplements vitamin E.
Bananas	Soften.
Borage oil	Taken as starflower, moisturises, softens and balances.
Cucumber	Cools, tones, refreshes, tightens.
Carrot oil, carrots	Good for scars and vitamin A production; antioxidant.
Egg white and yolk	White tightens and tones; yolk moisturises.
Evening primrose oil	Balances, softens, moisturises.
Frankincense essential oil	Promotes regeneration, regrowth and cell renewal.
Honey	Moisturises, softens.
Jojoba oil	Moisturises, soothes.
Lavender essential oil	Promotes soothing, regrowth, repair.
Lemon – fruit and essential oil	Bleaches, tones and tightens, soothes, deodorises.
Milk	Softens, soothes, moisturises – ass's milk is best!
Neroli essential oil	Tightens and soothes; great for stretch marks and skin cell regeneration.
Oatmeal	Exfoliates, provides vitamin E, soothes; antioxdant.
Olive oil	Softens and soothes, good for eczema; moisturises.

Rose water, essential oil	Encourages regrowth and regeneration; tonic and astringent.
Sweet almond oil	Provides vitamin E; moisturises.
Wheatgerm	Softens, provides vitamin E, soothes, exfoliates; antioxidant.
Water spritzes, sprays	Moisturise, invigorate, tone.

A final word on moisturisers. It's essential to keep your body as well as your face moisturised. Each time you bathe, wash, receive a treatment or carry out any of the body care treatments essential to the Water Detox programme, you should make sure you totally moisturise your entire body.

A daily skin care routine is essential if you wish your skin to stay in optimum condition. It is better to do it little and often. Every time you wash, simply follow with a moisturiser. If you get into the automatic habit of moisturising, then you won't have to think about it and you will begin to look wonderful in no time at all.

Keeping all your skin moisturised is important for detoxing. Keeping the cells and flesh in good condition will help to give the skin a warm glow, allow it to shed old dead cells more effectively and keep the flesh from looking dry and dull. Now we'll look at other ways of staying in fabulous all-over condition.

BEAUTY TOP TO TOE

Now we've seen how keeping the face and body moisturised is absolutely essential. But let's look at the inside story – nutrients for that special glow – and at how to keep an all-over polish.

Following a fabulously healthy diet packed full with hydrating foods will have you glowing from within and without. And if it's balanced and full of nutrients and antioxidants, this will maintain the equilibrium within your body as far as fluid and pH balance is concerned. Following the H_2O Nutrition Programme for just 18 days will make an amazing difference to your complexion and skin tone.

We have looked at what types of food we should be eating and how we can use water as our very own youth dew. Now we can look at ways to take care of our bodies to look just fab.

Feed Your Skin

There are many routes to great skin, but of course the two most important are diet and moisturising to protect. We have already looked at both. Now we need to look a bit closer at the antioxidants, vitamins, minerals and nutrients that help you grow and maintain wonderful skin.

A diet full of antioxidants will almost guarantee that your skin and body will stay younger for longer. Here are the star players.

Selenium
Selenium works to produce glutathione, which is a powerful antioxidant, detoxifying and protective. It is found in garlic, beans and lentils, onions and oily fish.

Vitamin A
Vitamin A comes in two forms, retinol and beta-carotene. It is said to keep our cells and tissues healthy. As such it will also keep our hair, teeth, bones and skin healthy and in optimum condition.

It is not difficult to get enough vitamin A in your diet because it is found in carrots, green vegetables and fish oils.

Vitamin C
Strong, healthy skin relies largely on vitamin C. We make collagen with vitamin C, and collagen, as I've shown, is responsible for keeping our skin plump and healthy. Vitamin C is found in green leafy vegetables – raw green vegetables are best. Citrus fruits, tomatoes and berries are also very high in vitamin C – crush the juice out, and hydrate.

Vitamin D
We can produce vitamin D, which is a natural skin tonic, when our skin is exposed to the sun, but unfortunately, exposing our skin to the

sun is not terribly good for us. We can therefore concentrate on eating the right foods to get enough. Oily fish is where you will find high concentration of vitamin D. And oily fish – salmon, sardines, mackerel and tuna – are all fully hydrating.

Vitamin E
Vitamin E protects our skin. It can also slow down the ageing process of our cells, most importantly skin cells. Some of the best sources for vitamin E are, surprisingly, broccoli, nuts and seeds, vegetable oils, sunflower and olive oils, and green vegetables. Needless to say, they are all part of the H_2O Nutrition Programme.

Thiamine
Found in sunflower seeds, thiamine is an important B vitamin, promoting good growth of skin cells.

Zinc
Essential for good skin and maintenance of great skin cells. Pumpkin seeds are a good source.

Calcium
Calcium is very important as it helps skin cells grow and develop. Great skin, nails, hair and teeth rely on good levels of calcium in our diets. A diet balanced in vitamin D is essential for full absorption of calcium. Green vegetables are high in calcium, as are salmon, water-cress, sunflower seeds, walnuts and sardines.

Water
As you definitely know by now, this is so, so, so important. Water keeps the skin, plump, hydrated and cleansed as it removes wastes from the body. A lack of water leads to dehydration, and dehydrated skin. Dehydrated skin becomes dry, wrinkly and pale. Putting creams on is no substitute for putting fluids in. Water is found in high concentration in fruits, fruit juices, vegetables and – I think you know what I am going to say – so drink up now.

So much for how the H_2O Nutrition Programme feeds our skin from the inside. Now we need to look at ways to look after our skin from the outside.

Dry Skin Brushing

In addition to keeping your body moisturised (see pages 105–9), you'll need to establish a regime of dry skin brushing every day for the whole 18-day programme. Dry skin brushing speeds up the lymph flow, which is the body's waste disposal system, and sloughs away any dead skin cells as well.

If you brush your skin every day, you will feel the benefits in just 3 or 4 days. The skin becomes soft and supple, and circulation is increased throughout the body. There really is nothing quite as effective for sloughing off dead skin cells, and invigorating the skin and circulation.

Dry skin brushing is also great for treating cellulite as it helps the body excrete waste and excess fluid.

It speeds up the efficiency of fluid flow between tissues, and prevents or reduces the pooling of fluid or water retention.

And it is extremely simple to do.

All you need is a bristle brush, a linen mitt, a dry flannel, or a towel. Just find something that has a mildly abrasive surface made of bristle or fabric.

You need to make sure that your skin is dry and that all the strokes you make flow upwards. Imagine you are trying to paint your body in big, sweeping brush strokes from your feet towards your head.

The strokes should be firm and rigorous, but slightly more gentle when working over more delicate skin: stomach, breast, backs of knees, armpits, and facial area. For the technique, see page 192–193.

Exfoliation

Exfoliation is the wet version of dry skin brushing. It sloughs off dead skin cells, leaving the skin soft and glowing.

There are hundreds of exfoliating products on the market, both natural and synthetic. Keep them in the shower and exfoliate on a regular basis – every 2 days is ideal for the body, and every 3 days, using a slightly lighter exfoliation product, is ideal for the face. Facial exfoliation should be done less often, as you don't want to overstimulate the sebaceous glands.

To exfoliate the body simply rub the product over your entire body in small circles, using firm strokes. Pay particular attention to areas of dry skin: elbows, knees, soles of feet. Once the exfoliation is complete, you should step into a warm shower or bath and continue rubbing until all of it is washed away.

Some homegrown exfoliating scrubs to try follow. Eating the food is beneficial, but we can absorb it through our skin as well!

Rice Polish

3 large tablespoons white rice – the only time white refined rice is appropriate on any detox programme

2 or 3 drops eucalyptus essential oil
1 pot natural yoghurt – this can be cow's, sheep's or goat's

Put the rice in a blender or coffee grinder or alternatively break down the grains in a pestle and mortar. Do not grind them too fine: they should still be quite coarse.

Mix the ground rice into a paste with half the yoghurt and the essential oil.

Massage the mix all over the body, avoiding the eyes and any broken or sensitive areas of skin. When the entire body has been covered with the mix, wash it off using firm strokes.

Once the mix has been washed away, smooth the remaining yoghurt all over. Leave it on for 5 minutes to moisturise and soften the skin, then rinse off.

Honey Body Smoother

2 large tablespoons sesame seeds
2 large tablespoons base or carrier oil of your choice

2 tablespoons honey – runny, not solid
2 drops lavender essential oil

Mix all the ingredients together in an ovenproof dish or pan. Heat the blend until warm, either on the hob or in the oven, or for just 15 seconds in the microwave. Check the temperature before scooping out the blend and rubbing it all over the body in firm, circular strokes.

Leave the blend on your body for at least 5 minutes, but don't get everything in your bathroom sticky!

Wash off with warm water, then pat dry with a warm towel.

Simple Salt Scrub

2 tablespoons natural sea salt for a rough scrub, or 2 tablespoons refined salt for a more gentle scrub

2 tablespoons carrier oil
2 drops juniper essential oil
2 drops ginger essential oil

Mix all the ingredients together in a bowl and then use as a scrub to exfoliate the entire body. This warming, relaxing and diuretic blend will speed up the flow of excess fluids. Leave on for 5 or 10 minutes, then rinse off.

Cleansing

There are great debates on how best to cleanse our skin. If you currently have a skin care regime that you are happy with, then you can just add a water cleanse to your current practice. If you don't, you may want to try the routine suggested in full, and then you will be able to see just how effective it is to take great care of your own skin.

Follow whatever normal skin care routine you have or, if you don't have one, when you have rinsed or washed you face, follow the next few steps:

- Splash your face with warm water at least 3 times.

- Splash your face with cold water at least 3 times.

- Pat the excess water from your skin with a towel; don't scrub it dry. It should still feel slightly damp.

- If your skin dries while you are dressing, spray a fine mist of water across your face and then apply your moisturiser immediately. You are trying to seal in a fine film of water on your skin's surface.

- Apply make-up as usual.

These few simple steps will give you glowing, rehydrated and protected skin in just a few days. You will hydrate from within and your skin will look plump and wrinkle-free, toned and fresh.

FIGHTING THE SKIN'S ENEMIES

Sunbathing

If your moisturiser contains an SPF of at least 15, it will not only protect your skin from moisture loss but will also protect it from the harmful and drying rays of the sun. Having a golden skin glowing with health does look good. Unfortunately, the appearance of a tan doesn't outweigh the damage and long-term ageing it causes. The importance of protecting our skin from the sun's harmful rays cannot be under-estimated. In fact, 80 per cent of wrinkles, dehydration, spots and colour blotches are due to premature ageing from sun damage.

Tans come and go in the fashion stakes, but in the realm of skin health they've always been a no-no. We may think that a tan is just a warm glow for fair skin and a dark honey colour for olive skin. It looks good, we say, and as long as we apply cream and then moisturise, the change in our skin is simply the time it takes for the colour to fade.

Not so. If you think of sailors or farmers or builders, or anyone who spends the day outside in the elements all year round, imagine their skin. Thick and leathery, it amply shows the rugged outdoor types they are. Well, if we expose our own skin to the elements we'll have it too.

Despite all this, we are very good at booking two weeks in the sun and going out on day one and bathing in the sun right the way through until check-in time. This fierce onslaught can only be totally damaging. Two weeks of healthy glow for several years of untold damage – not to mention the potential risk of skin cancers – is not much of a balance.

Unprotected skin will dry quicker, become leathery and hard, have small broken blood vessels near the surface, have blotchy and irregular pigmentation and look tired. And it will look old. Skin that has been out in the sun or exposed to the sun on a regular basis ages much quicker than skin that is protected from the elements. We can't just blame holiday sunbathing; we should protect our skin from dehydration and sun damage every time we go outside. Winter, with its cold winds and sleet, can be equally detrimental. UVA and UVB rays from the sun are the main culprits here. UVA and UVB rays age and burn, respectively. UVA will lead to dehydration, premature wrinkles, lines, and spots. UVB is the burning ray and also dries the skin and is believed to cause skin cancers.

We cannot avoid these rays, even on cloudy days, so it is important to make sure that your skin care regime includes a protective moisturiser or cream with at least 15 SPF. Smooth on the cream and see the visible signs of ageing gradually disappear.

Alcohol and Caffeine

We've had a look at how damaging alcohol and caffeine are generally, as they introduce toxins into the body. Alcohol is a drug that can kill in excess, although in the right amounts it can actually be beneficial. Red wine is packed with flavonoids that are antioxidant – they help the body reverse damage caused by free radicals and can help prevent the signs of ageing. Drinking the recommended 14 units for women and 21 for men per week is safe.

Caffeine is less extreme, but can also help to deplete the body of essential nutrients, to 'speed' us up in an unnatural manner and to make us dependent on the caffeine hit to function properly.

But how about their effects on the skin? The cartoon picture of a large-nosed, jolly old drinker with a foaming tankard is just how we could look if we drank to excess. The haggard black-coffee drinker nursing a bottle of whisky and cigarette late into the night might be an exaggeration, but one with a kernel of truth.

Regular drinking to excess causes the nose to swell, blood vessels to break and circulation to weaken. Pale skin, spots and dehydration are also almost certainly guaranteed. Caffeine will do the same, without the vein problems.

But that's not all. Alcohol and caffeine are diuretic and will make your body lose essential fluids, and they prevent the body from absorbing vitamins and minerals properly. So drinking more than a cup of coffee or 2 units of alcohol a day really shouldn't be part of your Water Detox beauty or health regime.

Cellulite

Cellulite involves an entire skin care regime of its own. Cellulite is also the only reason for actually trying to eliminate water during the Water Detox programme.

Cellulite is a build-up of toxins, retained water and waste products, characterised by bad skin texture. To get rid of it, you need to eliminate the excess, trapped fluids and the toxins, get the body to balance the flow of fluid, and improve skin tone to reach a state of optimum health. Detoxify, in short.

Female hormones don't actually cause cellulite, but they have a lot to do with it. This helps to explain why it is more likely to develop during puberty, pregnancy, and the menopause, whenever hormones are disrupted. In the same way, women who take hormone supplements such as the pill or HRT will also be altering their body's normal state and may prevent its ability to process fluids and lymph effectively and efficiently. That said, cellulite doesn't just disappear when hormonal shifts stop – unfortunately.

Everyone's body has fat cells. Hormones determine their size, distribution and accumulation. Stress, a sedentary lifestyle, posture, clothing, bad circulation and a dieting/bingeing cycle all contribute to the formation of cellulite.

When the circulation becomes sluggish, fats, slow-moving fluid and retained water collect between the connective tissues, resulting in cellulite. The appearance of cellulite varies. Some people talk of orange peel, others just see lumpy flesh, and sometimes you can hardly see it because the skin layers above are toned and healthy.

If we want to get rid of cellulite, we need to flush toxins out to cleanse the body and clear it. One of the reasons we retain fluid is because our bodies need it to survive. If we don't give the body enough water to flush and cleanse it, it will hold on to and retain as much as it can. If we don't have enough water in our bodies, we become dehydrated and the cleansing organs – the liver and kidneys – are not able to operate efficiently, and circulation becomes sluggish. It becomes a vicious circle. Excess fluid should be flushed out on a daily basis, and drinking 2 litres of water a day will do it.

You can therefore see that when you're fully hydrated, taking regular exercise, eating a good diet balanced in potassium and sodium, and practising a good skin and body care regime, you can reduce or reverse cellulite. Any product or treatment that stimulates lymph flow and manipulates flesh to aid detoxification and cleansing will speed up the process, as will hydrotherapy (see Chapter 3). But water is the key. Flushing out the body will speed up the process of banishing cellulite, and have hundreds of added benefits.

Now let's take a close look at what causes cellulite, so we can see how Water Detox combats it on all fronts.

Fluid retention

We retain fluid if our bodies are dehydrated.

The exchange of fluid in our cells is regulated by the content of sodium and potassium in our bodies. If we are dehydrated, the concentration of sodium in our cells rises and becomes too high to maintain a good operational balance. Our body attracts and holds more water, as the potassium content is not high enough to keep the exchange working efficiently.

The careful balance of sodium and potassium in the body is crucial to the efficient flow of oxygen, essential nutrients and waste to and from our cells. Sodium is found mainly inside our cells and potassium outside the cells. Essentially, the sodium/potassium balance within the body creates a fully functional pump – sodium absorbs fluids and potassium expels. If the pump is out of balance due to dehydration and a bad diet, then it is high in sodium – we absorb, but don't expel or cleanse efficiently. Once sodium becomes dominant, movement between cells becomes sluggish, the removal of waste slows down and leads to build-up, fluid is retained and congestion occurs.

The short-term effects are bloating and fluid retention; the long-term ones are bad cell renewal and regeneration. This will eventually mean irreversible damage to the internal structure of the cells. The Water Detox will prevent this from happening due to full hydration and a healthy, balanced diet.

Foods that encourage cellulite

All processed foods contain salt and we now know that salt causes water retention. We typically add salt when we cook and add more when the food reaches the plate. Our tastebuds have been so under-used that we need more salt than normal in order to eke out any flavour left in the processed foods. Our tastebuds also get used to salt and so we need a little more each time we taste.

It is much easier to grab foods full of salt than it is to grab foods bursting with potassium. This is found in large quantities in fresh fruits, fresh vegetables, sprouted beans, and seeds. You need to eat twice as much potassium as sodium in order to create a healthy flow of nutrients and efficient expulsion of waste. There are various ways to get the balance right:

- Avoid processed foods.

- Never add salt, when cooking, serving or eating.

- To get extra flavour in food, add herbs, spices and garlic instead of salt.

- Drain any tinned foods, especially fish, as these can be served in brine – salt water. Try to choose foods served in oils or water.

- Check the ingredient listings. Sodium, bicarbonate of soda, monosodium glutamate, sodium sulphite and sodium benzoate are all salt under a different name.

- Increase your potassium-rich food intake. Eat more vegetables such as carrots, broccoli, sprouts, cabbage and watercress.

- Increase your intake of seeds and beans – kidney, black beans, Aduki beans, and so on.

- Eat raw vegetables for more raw goodness. If raw doesn't suit, lightly grill, shallow fry, roast or stir fry. Keep the goodness in the food, not in the pan.

The not-so-convenient foods If you don't watch what you eat, just grab something to eat without even considering the implications, or eat mainly prepacked foods or ready meals, it is likely that your diet is high in salt, fats, and sugars. All of these ingredients are used to make foods taste nicer than they actually are. Then there are the colourings, flavourings, preservatives and sweeteners. There certainly won't be any antioxidants or essential nutrients.

When fats, sugars and salts are broken down by metabolism, much of the product is surplus to requirements – in short, there is very little nutrition left to benefit from. So what you get is largely fat and sodium. These are also the biggest causes of cellulite – sodium for water retention and fat for – well, fat.

In women cellulite travels to the thighs and buttocks – traditionally a place useful for protection and to support childbirth. The legacy is big thighs and a wobbly bottom.

Extra weight, or rapid weight gain or rapid weight loss, will put strain on the skin cells and tissue and eventually result in sagging, drooping and stretched flesh. If the flesh isn't totally hydrated, it can lead to lack of skin tone and decreased elasticity of the skin, and cellulite.

Yo-yoing disaster If you continually change the way you eat, one week eating plenty of food and the following eating practically nothing in order to balance the week before, your body will do everything to reduce the constant extremes of fluctuation. It is the same with water. If you drink a lot of water some weeks and then very little the next, your body will try to regulate itself by holding on to precious supplies.

We end up going into starvation mode. In order to regulate the peaks and troughs, the metabolism slows down in order not to burn fat. By doing so, it will then have fat stores to call upon next time we starve ourselves. The result is that even when dieting you don't lose weight because the body will not put itself in a position of jeopardy. Dehydration mode is the same: the body needs water, and if we don't give it enough it will keep up reserve stocks in order to function – resulting in fluid retention.

If you start to increase the quantities you eat and the fluid you drink over a short period of time, the body is not ready to deal with the overload. It is not in a position to automatically raise its metabolic or processing rate, so you feel bloated, your circulation and lymph system are overstretched, and you cannot process waste and fluid excess efficiently. The waste will then be stored in the body, mostly in areas such as the thighs and buttocks. Cellulite results, and the water is simply flushed out, so you spend all day just going to the toilet.

Eating regular meals of regular size and drinking the same amount of water on a regular basis will help the body to regulate itself.

Intolerances Personal food intolerances, if not addressed, can result in a build-up of substances that the body finds difficult to process. Many people have an intolerance to some very common foods. Their responses can range from simply feeling bloated after eating them to feeling sleepy, drugged or actually quite ill. We are not looking at actual allergies either – just foods that our bodies simply don't get on with. Here are a few of the main culprits:

• Dairy products

• Caffeine

• Alcohol

• Malt

• Maize

• Rye

• Refined flours

• Chocolate

- Yeast
- Wheat-based products
- Barley
- Refined sugar
- Refined starch

The easiest way to detect intolerance is to identify what you depend on in your diet or what you tend to crave on a regular basis. The foods you eat a lot of and eat regularly, such as bread or cheese, may be doing more harm than good and should be reduced or eliminated from your diet. If your body doesn't get on with them, don't spend time with them!

Inactivity

As we've learned, one of the main systems for processing waste in our bodies is called the lymph system. It doesn't have a pump or an automatic action; it relies entirely upon our hydration, muscle movement and gravity to push the lymph fluid around the body. If we sit still and don't move our muscles, it doesn't get to process as efficiently as it could if we were active. If we really don't move much over long periods, it can result in stagnation or pooling.

In any one day we typically spend eight hours lying down and eight hours sitting down. The remainder is split between standing and walking. We know that mobility is important in old or ill people in order to prevent muscle wastage, bed sores, weakness, oedema, bad circulation and poor respiration, but we never stop to think that any of these effects might happen to us through lack of movement. If it did it would be an extreme case, but if we don't take care our ankles can become bloated or our circulation sluggish just through our normal day-to-day existence.

Take a look at your daily activity levels. How many times do you sit down? How often do you take the car when you can walk? How often does your leisure activity include sitting or standing still? Change just one of these each day and you will notice the effects on your circulation almost immediately. Good circulation means efficient processing and elimination of waste, which in turn eliminates cellulite.

The skin and body care regime on your 18-day Water Detox addresses all the ways that can improve your cellulite – and may just wash it clean away. Make sure you follow it correctly for every one of the 18 days, and I personally guarantee great results.

7

Healing Waters

WATER IS NOT ONLY A CLEANSER. It is also an internal healer. In this section you will be able to see the power of water as medicine. Many common niggles and complaints can be solved or eased by simply drinking more water. Many more serious illnesses that are caused by dehydration can be cured by drinking water, and many illnesses can be prevented by allowing the body to work at optimum hydration and full immunity.

Take 2 litres of water per day, just as the doctor ordered.

The human body is 75 per cent water. If our bodies maintain this percentage, they can operate quite healthily and efficiently. We can compare this to our cars. If we have oil in the tank, everything works well and efficiently and we don't give it a second thought. If the oil levels drop, the car simply stops. This doesn't happen often because we have a gauge in the car that flashes when levels are low and we also have a dipstick to do a physical check. Despite these indicators we can still run out of oil, so it is not perfect; but at least we know for a fact that it is damaging. It is exactly the same for the body. If we don't manage 75 per cent hydration, things don't work as well, and if the levels get too low we stop functioning properly. Dehydration is dangerous and unhealthy. Unfortunately, we don't have a dipstick or a flashing light. What we do have is skin tone and aches and pains. They are the first indicators that everything is not hydrated in our bodies.

We also know that the liver, kidneys, lymph system, circulation, lungs and cells all rely on a very high-percentage water content. These organs are about cleansing and flushing toxins through the body. We cannot wash and cleanse without splashing excess amounts of water around the bathroom or kitchen, so why should our bodies be able to? Whatever the truth and however logical the logic, we still don't drink enough water to keep our bodies' water levels optimum.

We expect the body to remain healthy but we don't keep it lubricated and efficient. One of the simplest ways to see that we need water for health is the fact that water helps to balance the pH in our bodies. That is to say, it balances the acid and alkaline levels.

The ideal level of pH in the body is between 7.4 and 7.5, which is slightly alkaline. If we are dehydrated and develop a pH balance below 7.4, we become too acidic, stressed and tired, our blood becomes sluggish and we can develop high blood pressure. Eventually, too much acidity can cause death.

We should eat a diet rich in alkaline-forming foods and drink enough water to prevent dehydration. If we dehydrate then the body becomes too acidic. Our bodies simply cannot be healthy if we are constantly too acidic, as this causes:

- Ulcers

- Gas

- Irritable bowel

- High blood pressure

- Constipation

- Heartburn

- Indigestion

It is no mistake that pure water has a pH balance of 7.4, perfect for keeping the body hydrated and in balance. So these common conditions can be greatly improved with a simple glass of water.

It is no mistake that I'm asking you to give up coffee for the 18 days, as it actively increases acidity in the body!

There are many foods that can also keep the balance of pH in the blood at a constant level of 7.4 to 7.5. All of these foods feature heavily on the H_2O diet.

Think in terms of a flowing river – everything clear and sparkling, cleansing everything as it runs by. It will discard anything that falls in by depositing it along the bank later on its journey. If something gets in the way of the flow, it immediately, almost instantaneously, finds a way around the problem; and the water is renewed on a regular basis so nothing can be harboured in the depths. The water is fresh and pure. If we stumble across a mountain spring, we naturally gravitate towards it and either swim or paddle in it or drink it.

If our bodies are at full and optimum hydration then we are like a flowing river, negotiating every illness, infection, ache and pain. We find a way to wash away the symptoms and to go around the cause.

If you think in terms of a stagnant pond with green slime on top, you can imagine that if the body gets anywhere near this state it certainly isn't ideal. Things start to slow down, the body begins to feel sluggish, and there isn't enough fluid or flow for it to get better. Stagnant water is also a prime condition for the spread of germs. Moist conditions can harbour some of the simplest but most damaging germs. You would never even consider paddling in stagnant water because the immediate response, if it doesn't smell, is that it is unhealthy, and you just don't know what is harboured under the surface or what is growing in it. Some of the most dangerous diseases we have in this world are waterborne.

So why do we let our bodies spend so much time nearer to stagnancy than full hydration? Why do we let the body struggle to stay healthy, doing the best it can to pull on the reserves it has? All we need to do is drink 2 litres of water a day to see how hydrated and healthy we become. Little things like lower back pain and joint aches will quite literally be washed away. More serious back pain will be alleviated as the water supports our skeleton. Skin conditions are flushed out and the most impressive of all is that our immune system can fight with every tool in the box if we keep our cells fully hydrated. A simple glass of water every hour, and we can help prevent, delay and combat every minor and major illness we get or are subjected to.

Bear in mind the facts we discussed at the start of the book. They are worth repeating:

- Our brain is 75 per cent water.
- Blood is 92 per cent water.
- Bones are 22 per cent water.
- Muscles are 75 per cent water.
- Brain cells are 82 per cent water.
- Moderate dehydration can cause headaches and even dizziness.
- Our brains weigh 1.5 kilogrammes, of which 200 grammes are actual brain and the rest is water.
- We need water to exhale.
- Water inside the body regulates our body temperature.
- Water inside the body maintains the pH balance of the body – the acidity and alkalinity.
- Water helps us to breathe as it moistens air on inhalation.
- Water helps remove toxins and waste.
- On hot days, sweating causes us to lose up to 16 glasses of water per day.
- 2 out of 3 people drink the recommended minimum of 8 glasses of water a day.
- Thirst indicates a state of dehydration.
- Not drinking enough water can result in dry and itchy skin, feelings of tiredness and lethargy upon waking, and tiredness during the day.
- Long-term dehydration causes high blood pressure, bad circulation, bad digestion, poor kidney function, and slow bodily operation and processing.
- The body needs as much water in cold weather as it does in hot weather.
- Mild dehydration slows down metabolism by as much as 3 per cent.

We become dehydrated when our water levels are down by just 2 per cent. It really is so easy to be dehydrated – but it is even easier to be fully hydrated.

WATER AND COMMON AILMENTS

Water makes sense to me, because I know that when I drink it I feel so much better, and when I fall off the wagon and my fluid intake consists of coffee and alcohol with a few glasses of water, I know how tired I get and how I should get back up to optimum fluid levels.

Then I read a book called *Your Body's Many Cries for Water*, by F. Batmanghelidj. It was the final piece in the jigsaw. Someone had done research and had experience of how water wasn't just good for you in a general way – general wellbeing, general health levels – but that it is actually a medicine.

We've seen how 'taking the waters' is an age-old process. The ancient Roman baths, the Dead Sea, Sebastian Kneipp, and all the other aspects of how valuable water is to total wellbeing have all been discussed. But the cherry on the top, the icing on the cake, the facts to support the argument – if I had left you in any doubt by this stage – can all be seen in Dr Batmanghelidj's work.

And water is not dangerous as long as we stick to safe amounts. Two litres a day over the period of the day is totally safe, but 2 litres in an hour can make us feel weak and debilitated, as we can actually 'flood' or drown our bodies from the inside. If you drink too quickly in extreme circumstances you can prevent the body from correct absorption of minerals and salts – but you really would have to be drinking huge amounts in a very short space of time.

The following descriptions are based on the findings of Dr Batmanghelidj. Follow the suggestions to see if your symptoms are alleviated. What I cannot say is that they are a total cure. Take the advice but, if the symptoms persist or you continue to feel unwell, you should consult your medical practitioner for further diagnoses.

Arthritis

If we are dehydrated, the fluid sacs in our joints dry up and can no longer protect and cushion our joints. We know by now that our blood circulation relies on water, our cells rely on water and so do our bones. If we don't drink sufficient water, the blood becomes sticky. Our circulation becomes sluggish. Our bones dry out a little and cause friction, and the sacs of fluid that normally protect the joints and cushion every move we make no longer work as well as they should.

We will feel pain, the contact between joints and the lack of protection between bones will mean the body will keep us warned of the dangers. We 'read' pain as something being wrong, so we make doctors' appointments. If we were to read pain in joints, and aches and irritations, as the first signs of dehydration, then we could drink more water immediately and see if the problem goes away. If it doesn't, then it is obviously necessary to take further measures. But you can always increase your water intake while waiting for your appointment.

High Blood Pressure and Heart Conditions

If we become dehydrated, our blood becomes dehydrated too. If we have insufficient levels of water in our body or higher levels of stimulants like alcohol and caffeine, the blood can get sluggish and fail to flow as freely as it should. The blood then reaches organs and limbs, etc., less efficiently, which can cause problems for blood pressure regulation, heart regulation and heart stress.

Why is this? The heart is a pump that maintains our circulation and most of our bodily functions are regulated by it. If the fluid it pumps changes state or content, it is put under more stress, or altered, neither of which is favourable. Drinking the correct fluid levels ensures that the body maintains an optimum operating environment. If the problems still continue, you will have weeded out simple dehydration as a cause.

Excess Weight

There are figures from the US that suggest 75 per cent of all hunger pangs are actually sensations of thirst. When we get hungry our first response should be to drink a glass of water. Drinking water will determine if you really were hungry or if you were actually thirsty all along. Take a large glass of water 30 minutes before you sit down to eat, and don't drink with your meal. Make sure your meal is made up entirely of foods from the H_2O Nutrition Programme, and you shouldn't feel thirsty during your meal.

So you may not actually be hungry; you could just be very, very thirsty.

Asthma and Allergies

Asthma and allergies are irritated or made worse when the level of toxins in the body becomes too high or too concentrated. Drinking more fluid will help to dilute these concentrations to prevent them getting to the dangerous levels that the allergy or asthma cannot handle. Using water to cleanse the system will keep the dilutions manageable and may just enable the sufferer to reduce the amount of drugs they are taking after close, professional monitoring.

Back Pain

Our spine is supported and cushioned by sacs of fluid between each vertebra – discs. Each of these discs supports our day-to-day movement and impact. We exercise and jump up and down, causing the discs to cushion any joints from damage or shock. If the fluid levels in the body are low, the fluid levels in the spinal column may be reduced. Think of bouncing on a space hopper; if you remove the space hopper then there is no bounce, but instead more of a horrible jolting thud which at best is extremely painful and at worst is actually paralysing if the impact is taken through the disc to the spinal column and the nerves.

In general, if you get lower back pain or aching joints, drink more water in the first instance and see if you can feel the support you need.

Dyspepsia, Heartburn and Indigestion

We talked at the start of this chapter about the damage acid can do to our bodies. If we become dehydrated, the pH balance is disrupted and the acidity of the body is increased. This acidity can have an impact on the fluid in our cells. In the case of heartburn or indigestion it shows that the stomach lining has become dehydrated and is no longer protecting the stomach from the strong digestive acids it contains. Drinking water to maintain full hydration means prevention. And if the symptoms do occur, drinking water slowly over a period of time will help.

Below are suggestions for relieving the symptoms of some of the very common ailments and also some of the less frequent illnesses. You should by now be drinking your full quota, so these are ways to alleviate pain and discomfort. If you have not reached your full water quota by now, then what can I say ...

Arthritis We have spoken about the water intake for arthritis, but there are also ways in which you can relieve pain from the outside, including steamroom, sauna, or flotation to alleviate pressure.

Back pain Flotation to alleviate pressure. Thalassotherapy for mineral intake and relaxation. Watsu to free the joints.

Colds Inhalations, steaming the cold, compresses, bathing in oils, thermotherapy/hydrotherapy.

Circulation Dry skin brushing, thermotherapy/hydrotherapy. Ginger baths and thalassotherapy.

Constipation Sitz baths, hydrotherapy/thermotherapy. Epsom salts baths.

Cystitis Warm baths with juniper or tea tree oil. Drinking at least 350 millilitres of water per hour to flush the infection away.

Headaches Hydrotherapy concentrating on the forehead and back of the neck. Lavender applied in steamrooms, and compresses.

Stress Body-temperature bathing and then hydrotherapy. Flotation to help process and eliminate negative thoughts and images.

Pain relief Cold application, cold compress, ice packs.

From this point forwards, if you are feeling tired, or maybe a little nauseated, drink a glass of water and follow up in half an hour with another – and see how you feel.

If you are aching and your joints are sore, take the same medicine – a glass of water and then half an hour later, another one.

Use water as your first-base medicine. Once your body is hydrated you can get a better picture of how you are truly feeling. It is no coincidence that hospitals feed fluids into the body almost as soon as you are admitted for serious illnesses. They need you to be hydrated so that your chances of recovery are enhanced. I once spoke to a senior nurse in a psychiatric ward who told me that most of her patients were severely dehydrated upon admission. The first job they need to do is to rehydrate before they can get the real picture.

So, take the advice: rehydrate as the first step in your diagnosis.

8

Go with the Flow

W E'VE BEEN TALKING MAINLY about the body so far, but
water can be used to detox many other aspects of our lives.
Water can help cleanse our minds of negative thoughts,
and clear up emotions or feelings that distress or upset us. Taking a
warming bath is truly wonderful, but being able to use the water in our
life and in our body to calm our own waters inside is essential to
achieve total balance.

We can be wonderfully hydrated and physically fit with glowing
skin and bags of energy, but if we don't feel positive about ourselves or
our life for some reason then we won't feel totally detoxed. Getting rid
of negative or destructive influences and sad and unhappy thoughts is
an essential part of the Water Detox. During the 18-day programme
you will be harnessing the energy of the water in your life and seeing
how you can use it to your best advantage and time it for optimum
results. Feel the force!

- **The power of the moon** You should get a diary or moon chart that
  tells you dates for the phases of the moon, and you should start your

programme 3 days before a full moon. You must map your behaviour, emotions and feelings against the cycles of the moon.

- **Feng Shui for wealth** During the 18-day programme, you should determine the good and bad water in your life and cleanse the flow. Follow the section on Feng Shui and clear the way for free flow.

- **Feel the vibration** You should check the level of electromagnetic fields in your life and get them to a level that doesn't disrupt or harm you.

- **Read the signs** Check your star sign and those of your friends to increase your knowledge about yourself and those close to you.

- **Water medicine** You should take some water medicine in the form of homeopathy, flower remedies, crystal elixirs or animal medicine.

- **Relax and destress** Use the vibrational pull of your waters to get you in or out of a mood.

You will be empowering your inner waters and your life.

Hydration isn't the whole story. The water content of our bodies can affect us in many different ways. We can also affect the water we put into our bodies in many ways.

In fact, we are totally affected by water and we can totally affect water. The next section explores just a few of the amazing ways in which we should consider water as part of our lives – ways that can make sense of things, help things and be used to change us. Water isn't just for drinking, cleansing and swimming in. That is just the start of it.

Water is affected by electricity – as we know, it conducts it extremely efficiently. Water is affected by vibration and resonance – the ripples on a pond from the sinking pebble or the sound of a car backfiring. Water can be changed in a second when subjected to any of these forces.

And water changes us when we are subjected to its forces, its resonance, and its vibration. Why, after all, spend so much of our time searching it out or exploring it? It has an effect on us, and we never question it. It is almost addictive as a source of relaxation, but we never really ask why.

GOING TO THE WATER

When we go on holiday, we go to rest and recuperate, to invigorate and energise, and to 'get away from it all'.

If you browse through the holiday brochures, what is the single most featured item in the pictures? Water. It features on every page of the holiday brochures in varying colours of blues and greens and in various states: sea, lake, snow, spa, pool, and so on.

Sailing, canoeing, windsurfing, skiing, snowboarding, ice skating, waterskiing, diving, snorkelling, cruising, white-water rafting, walking along the sea shore, river's edge or canalside, taking barge trips, going to spas and lakes, gazing at fountains and waterfalls. Anywhere and everywhere in the world – but the one certain thing is that when we go on holiday we go to the water.

The reason we do this is because we enjoy the properties of water, feel its effects, enjoy looking at it, and still have no clue as to the real and profound effect it is actually having on us. We just know that we have had a holiday and we feel ready to come back and face the world after our short or long break.

The fact is that by spending time near water we feel ourselves reach a balance and become calmer. If we spend time near water we can feel refreshed or invigorated, depending on the type of water. Remember, we are made of water, so the energy or vibe of the water we are near will be the energy or vibe we experience.

Crashing waves and white-water rafting water are energetic, exhilarated water – we become energised and exhilarated even just looking at it.

Millponds and trickling streams are calm and relaxed water – we listen to the simple sounds of this water and become more relaxed.

We recently held a sweat lodge in Surrey, England. The purpose of sweat lodges is to go through a spiritual cleansing and to emerge from the lodge purified and renewed in both energy and spirit. The sweat lodge is built for the purpose and the participants join inside in a day of singing, praying and sweating for total cleansing. Sweat lodges are traditional Native American in origin, but steam has been used for cleansing for hundreds of years in Russia, Japan and Africa. We use saunas for a similar purpose – to cleanse away the toxins through extreme heat and sweat. Not quite as spiritual as the sweat lodge, but along the same principles.

The Native American shaman who was hosting our lodge sent word that no one could take part if they were on their 'moon time' – that is, menstruating. This started my interest in the significance of the moon and its effects on the earth, the human body, and spiritual ceremonies.

THE POWER OF THE MOON

The moon has long been known as a powerful and mysterious force. Even if we don't believe in any of its mystical qualities, we are very much aware of the moon's different stages. We will also certainly be able to blame any strange behaviour or events on its being a full moon – remember that the word 'lunatic' refers to the moon's ancient name, Luna.

So what is the actual power of the moon, and what is its relevance to the Water Detox? As I've said elsewhere in this book, the moon is responsible for tides around the world. The gravitational pull of the earth's waters is due to the positioning of the moon. As well as tidal waters, this gravity will also pull at any other water on the earth. Remember, we're three-quarters water – so the moon will also have a significant effect on us, emotional and physical. Our water will also be pulled to varying degrees at different times of the moon cycle/month. It is for this reason that the mythology of people changing emotionally and mentally during the moon's phases begins to become not a myth, but a very practical fact.

If you understand the moon's role in your life, you start to map it against your own physical and emotional ups and downs. Then, it may just be that you can see reflections of the highs and lows you experience.

Not only does the moon affect water on earth and water within our bodies; it also has effects on weather systems and other terrestrial phenomena. Rain, volcanic action, earthquakes, hurricanes, and many other extreme weather conditions are greatly affected by the pull of the moon.

To understand just how the moon affects water, and how much of a science this actually is, you have to grasp the basics of the relationship between the sun, moon and earth.

The earth orbits the sun every 364.25 days. As the earth moves around the sun, it also spins on its own axis, with a total revolution taking 24 hours. It takes 29.5 days for the moon to orbit the earth.

You can start to see that our calendar is based on these timings:

- The duration of our year is 364.25 days – the time the earth takes to orbit the sun.

- The duration of our calendar month is between 30 and 31 days – and it takes 29.5 days for the moon to orbit the earth. The word 'moon' is the origin of the word 'month'.

- The duration of our day is 24 hours – and it takes 24 hours for the earth to make one complete turn on its axis.

The planets work in perfect harmony and we have taken the timings for our everyday lives from these movements. Our days, months and years are all dictated by the time it takes for the movements of the planets. We are therefore already working in time to the relationships between moon, sun and earth.

The earth measures 19,320 kilometres across, the moon just 3,494 kilometres across. This means that the moon's gravitational pull on the earth is about one-sixth of the earth's on the moon – still enough to have a quite profound effect on the earth's waters, crops and harvests, and weather systems. As we are looking at gravitational pull, we can also see that the moon has an equally profound effect on the electromagnetic field of the earth, and enough to have a quite profound impact on us as well. You only need to think of the effect that putting two magnets together can have on their immediate fields.

As well as the everyday effect of the moon on the earth, there are also times when this is greatly enhanced, when the moon and sun are aligned and pulling together on the earth's gravity.

The most tangible way to see how the moon affects us is to look at the tidal charts for any coastline, anywhere in the world. Every single day there are high and low tides and these are directly and totally aligned to the position of the moon, the sun and the earth. The point where the surface of the earth is facing the surface of the moon will have a high tide. Here, the moon is pulling the water towards its own gravitational force. In the areas where the water is being pulled away, low tide occurs. The tides happen twice a day, 2 low tides and 2 high tides, anywhere and everywhere in the world. The effect of the moon on earth's waters is constant.

So it follows that the water within our bodies must be affected in a very similar way. There will be constantly changing tides within our own bodies. We will respond to the gravitational pull of the moon, in terms of our water content.

Our year is made up of what we refer to as lunar months. There are 12 each year, and in each month there is a full cycle of the moon – a full orbit of the moon around the earth. During this month-long period, the moon is new, full, waxing and waning. The cycle repeats continually as the moon circles the earth.

You can use the lunar cycle to affect your own tides. You can see below that if you are making changes in your life or wishing to bring something to a close, the moon allows a time and a place for everything. Match these times and you can use its power to strengthen your actions and bolster your confidence.

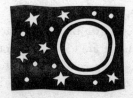

Phase	A good time for ...
New moon	Planning and preparation. The new moon is about preparing for a new beginning.
Full moon	Creativity and strength, being fruitful and productive. You are firing on all cylinders, getting things done and being effective. This is the time for creation.
Waning moon	Closure, finishing projects. Bringing things and issues to a conclusion.
Dark moon	Meditation, contemplation and mystery – the 'dark side'.

The New Moon

With the new moon, the right-hand side of the moon is illuminated. The ends of the crescents are pointing to the left. The moon is called 'new' until half of it is illuminated on the right-hand side.

The new moon is the start of the month or of a cycle. New moons are used to clear what has gone before and to move forward.

This phase is the first three days of the new cycle. It is a time to plan, prepare and think ahead, to start new projects, to concentrate on your own growth and development and your own personal health.

The Full Moon

After the new moon, we move towards the full moon. Over days the illumination spreads from the right-hand side over the whole surface of the moon that faces us.

The full moon is a very exciting time. It denotes full fertility and ripeness, and anyone trying to conceive would be well advised to concentrate their efforts during the full moon and the days leading up to it. Look at the full moon and see how like an egg it looks. This will help you to remember to take advantage, or be very wary! The full moon is the time of fertility. I once visited an astronomer and he warned me that if I was trying to become pregnant (I wasn't!), I should spend the full moon time holding babies and in the company of young children and pregnant women. Needless to say, I wouldn't touch any baby offered to me and cancelled my invitation to a christening!

The time of the full moon is also when women are at their most powerful and most creative because the power of the moon is strongest and most potent. You should draw on 'Mother Moon' if you need help or support in any area of your life at the time of the full moon. The Western medical world is also beginning to think that there is sufficient evidence to suggest that any woman needing a breast operation or any major gynaecological procedure will have a greater chance of a full and speedier recovery if the operation takes place in this time – they do not relate it to the moon but to the woman's ovulation cycle. It is interesting that something our forefathers probably took for granted has now been considered as valuable information for the knowledgeable and sometimes arrogant Western world.

As it is the most powerful time, it is also the time of the greatest impact. Remember the Luna/lunacy connection? Crimes committed during a full moon are treated more leniently in some parts of the world, as are crimes committed during certain types of weather. The winds in Spain are reported to bring madness to residents of the area. For this reason, the fault of the crime does not lie entirely at the perpetrator's door!

If you are aware that the moon has an influence on your moods, you will be only too familiar with the changes that occur. You can feel emotionally or mentally unstable, you may be more prone to making mistakes or having accidents, or more things may go wrong in your life. If this is the case, just check to see the phase of the moon, and I can guarantee that the full glow of this beautiful satellite will be looking down on you.

The Waning Moon and the Dark Phase

You can see the moon wane as the light begins to fade from the right-hand side until only the left-hand side is illuminated, and the ends of both crescents are visibly pointing to the right.

The waning moon is the end of the cycle, the time to finish things that need to be concluded or to close a door that was left open.

After the moon has waned, it is the time for the darkness that brings us full cycle to the next new moon. This darkness is the time for mystery, for contemplation, and for discarding anything you wish to leave behind before entering the new cycle and new, fresh beginnings.

To end something or to close something needs thought and consideration. This phase of the moon is therefore suited to activities such as meditation, thought, and contemplation.

The Female Moon

Moon energy is feminine, and the energy of the sun is masculine. We call the earth 'Mother Earth' and we call the sky 'Father Sky'.

The sun means day, hot and bright, which in Chinese terms we call *yang* energy. It is fast, hot and feeds the earth. It is light, and associated with action and masculinity.

Moon energy is dark and mysterious, cold and quiet. In Chinese medicine, these qualities are called *yin* energy.

Together the *yin* and *yang* of the moon and sun complement each other perfectly. We need the heat of the day to grow the crops and give light. We need the sun to nourish the plants and seeds. The moon is dark and restful and germinates the seeds and helps the nurturing and growth of the plants.

The female aspects of the moon are worth thinking about. The cycle of the moon is directly aligned to the female menstrual cycle – the word *men* is Latin for 'moon', and the word 'menstrual' is from the same Latin origin. Just as we discussed earlier, a woman is at her most fertile during a full moon and the days leading up to it. As women ovulate they become creative; they are, after all, creating life. At the time women menstruate, they cast away the unused egg in order to start again – the cycle repeats itself. At this time the female is at her most perceptive and powerful. So much so that many religions, ancient civilisations and native tribes chose to separate the menstruating female from the other members of the tribe or family.

At this time, a woman's influence or spiritual powers were thought to be so consuming and powerful that they could disrupt any ritual or ceremony.

On a final note …

Once in a Blue Moon ...

If something is rare, or rarely happens, we say it happens 'once in a blue moon,' but even though I have said this a million times it wasn't until quite recently that I heard on the radio that it is based on fact.

A 'blue moon' is a month when there are two full moons. This can happen in a long 31-day month. The rarity of this occurrence makes the potency quite phenomenal. The first moon is quite normal, but the second, 'extra' moon is the potent empowering one. The effect on the tides and the earth's water are increased and dramatic tidal readings, volcanic actions and extreme weather conditions are most likely to occur at these times. Blue moons don't often happen but when they do – watch out!

In fact, use a blue moon to make big plans, to sow the seeds for your future. You must be careful what you wish for on a blue moon – it might just come true ...

Once you have seen how water can empower you, you can now begin to see how it can increase flow around you. A flow of wealth, a wealth of health, a wealth of emotions and a wealth of total wellbeing.

FENG SHUI AND WATER

And in the Chinese science of Feng Shui, money is represented by water.

We always talk about 'cash flow' – either it is not flowing or it flows in and then out just as quickly! We talk about 'increasing the flow' when what we are meaning is that we wish to earn more. According to Feng Shui laws, wherever we place water or have water in our home or life will dictate how wealthy and healthy we are. If it is in the wrong place neither wealth nor health will flow easily, while if it is in the right place it can bring great wealth and fabulous fitness. The Water Detox follows some simple guidelines of Feng Shui and can increase both your wealth and your fitness. Get into free flow!!

The impression seems to be that we give money some 'watery' qualities. It flows freely. We can also look at techniques to prevent the flow from turning into a trickle or positively cascading out of our lives before we are able to get it to work for us or invest it!

One of the largest investments we make or largest outlays we have is our mortgage or rent. We spend huge amounts of our incomes on our homes and dwellings. It is in our culture to spend large amounts of time making our day-to-day living more enjoyable. The DIY boom is testament to this.

But do we ever think about our homes actually making money for us? Or, actually tangibly, being able to improve the quality of our lives, and not just by sitting in them or coming home to them?

In this section, we are going to look at ways in which we can help our homes to actually earn money or increase our health and wealth for us – and not by selling them.

It is no secret that the most popular television programmes at the moment are the makeover programmes, whether personal, home decoration, or garden design. We are actively taking an interest in developing our surroundings to make us feel good and 'at home'.

There are many other cultures that attach a little more importance to their surroundings. In Tibet and Vietnam they follow Phong Thuy, in the Philippines, Indonesia and Thailand they follow Hong Sui and in Japan, Hawaii and India they believe in Vaastu Shastra. It is unlikely that you have heard of any of these disciplines. Vaastu Shastra is potentially the only one you might find in a book. But it's very likely you will have heard of Feng Shui.

The Chinese use the rules and science of Feng Shui (actually pronounced 'fung shway' or 'fung shoy') throughout the world due to interest from Western cultures. Its popularity stems from our increasing desire to get the best out of our homes and, more importantly, to become happier, healthier and wealthier individuals. It seems to be entirely British that we shouldn't admit to wanting to make money and be successful. Feng Shui allows this, and supports the desire to make the most of what we have got.

The two Chinese characters Feng and Shui literally mean 'wind' and 'water'. This shows that Feng Shui is concerned with earthly, not spiritual, influences. Feng Shui is not a religion. It is not an art. But it is a science; there are strict rules of application and along with the overall philosophy there are many, many tools, techniques and exercises to be used when introducing its principles into your life.

Simply put, Feng Shui is about getting all the positive energy available to you into your life, keeping it there, and using it to its optimum, and then allowing all negative energy a free route out of your life. Keeping up a constant flow of good energy without any blockages will bring health, wealth and prosperity – something we could all do with more of.

There are many schools of Feng Shui. To dictate the school you should follow would be arrogant of me, but there are many, many books and magazines that you can read to find out the basics.

It is not always totally necessary to employ a consultant before you use Feng Shui in your life. If you read about the subject as much as you can, you will be able to see that some smaller projects can be under-taken by yourself with the help of a good book. If you want to make some big changes – and I don't necessarily mean big structurally, but big in significance – you would be well advised to find a qualified and recommended consultant. They will invariably know the specific things to concentrate on so you don't waste your time on irrelevant work.

How do you set about finding the right consultant for you? They can be very expensive, but if you get a fully qualified practitioner who has studied for many years rather than done a few weekend courses you will find that the results of the consultation will undoubtedly be worth the initial outlay. (See page 196 for recommended addresses.)

Alternatively, you could write to a local school of Feng Shui and volunteer as a practice client for a student completing their studies.

While you are deciding how to introduce water Feng Shui into your life, there are some simple tools for you to use that can start you on your journey of increasing the flow of wealth through your life and home or workplace.

The Five Elements

When you study Feng Shui, one of the first things you will be introduced to are the five elements. Everything and everyone in our lives has an element. Some have more than one, but everything has a main, dominant or 'big' element. These are:

- Water
- Metal
- Earth
- Fire
- Wood

Each of these elements has a supporting relationship with one of the others, and some of them have a destructive relationship with the other elements. See below for examples.

Supportive cycle

Fire supports Earth
When fires burn they produce ash. Ash is highly nutritious to the earth, and adding it to the earth will increase the earth's nutrients.

Earth supports Metal
The metal oxides and ores bond together to form metals, both precious and common, deep inside the earth. In this way the earth 'grows' metal.

Metal supports Water
When metal is melted it flows like water. Water is produced by metal.

Water supports Wood
If we water plants and trees, they can grow and prosper. Water supports wood in this way.

Controlling cycle

Fire controls Metal
If fire burns hot it can melt metal. Fire is destructive of metal.

Earth controls Water
If we throw earth into water it becomes muddied and dirty and undrinkable. Earth destroys water in this way.

Metal controls Wood
Metal implements such as saws and axes can chop down trees and chop up wood. Metal destroys wood.

Water controls Fire
Water is used to put out a fire.

As you can see, there are combinations of the elements that are more productive than others. If you are studying Feng Shui seriously, you soon begin to see that you need to have a deep understanding of the elements, their relationships, and their potential, and then you have to have an equally deep understanding of the element of the object or person you are trying to affect.

The facts of our birth play a key role here. Each of us has an hour, a day, a month, and a year of birth. Each of these dates and times has a very certain element and it is these elements that determine our futures and our lives. Knowing this information and all the associated information gives us the key to know or find out about every aspect of our lives, in the past, present and most definitely the future.

The elements also have compass points aligned to them. The element water is the north, and can be represented by the *yang* colour black and the *yin* colour blue – dark blue.

Every aspect has a *yang* and *yin* aspect, or a male and female aspect.

As we said earlier, Feng Shui has a lot to do with the flow of energy. In order for energy to flow, it needs to have all blockages or obstacles removed. Anything controlling should be looked at, and anything supporting should be encouraged. Anything that would shut it off or redirect it or prevent it from entering every aspect of your home should be rectified. In the same way, anything that speeds up the energy or contributes to too much energy should also be carefully looked at so that a balanced flow is maintained.

One of the first things you can do as a personal exercise is to imagine that you, yourself, are free-flowing energy. If this is difficult, then imagine you are a fine mist that can get into every nook and niche. Now, stand outside your house on the street and face your front door and imagine that you are the positive energy or the mist.

Look around you and begin to judge if there is anything that is preventing your easy access to your home. Is there a tree across your front door? Is your front door old and dirty? Is the drive long and funnel-like so that you use too much energy speeding up towards the door and overpowering it, or is the path just long enough for the energy to arrive at the door ready for entry?

Does the front door work, or does it stick? Does your hallway lead you through the house, or is there a wall in the way that blocks the flow? Is there a door you never use or that is blocked by a piece of furniture? If so, clear the blockage and open the door – let the energy flow in. Have you got mirrors facing each other? As a rule, that just bounces energy back and forwards and is disruptive and interferes with the flow, so move the mirrors so that they don't reflect each other but reflect the energy out into the house and encourage its path. Hang all doors so that they open into the rooms and not back out into the hall or corridor so that when you approach a room you naturally flow into it.

Check that the back door is not blocked and opens outwards so that all energy, once it has passed through the house and has been used, can then exit freely. Check, however, that the front door is not in line with the back door as you will find energy entering your home and then zooming straight out of the back of your property before it gets to circulate its beneficial properties.

Check for clutter or rubbish. If something would trip you up or get in your way, then think of it metaphorically. Is there stuff in your life that trips you up or catches you out? If so, clear it up.

Once you have completed your journey through the house, you will be more aware of your home dynamics and may wish to make some changes to get the optimum flow. You can now get down to some water specifics. If the flow of water represents the flow of wealth, do we have any dripping taps or leaking pipes that may be wasting money? Do you have any pools, ponds, streams or rivers that have been having a profound effect on your life without you knowing it and are you thinking of installing an indoor pool in the place that positively encourages the water to flow *away* freely out of your life?

One of the first things that some people say when you mention Feng Shui is a jokey 'Oh no! I've forgotten to put the loo lid down, all my money is escaping down the pan.' Well, smile sweetly and tell them just how accurate they are and that you didn't know they were such advanced students of Feng Shui!

Seriously, there is a lot to the toilet water theory. If water is wealth, then leaving the toilet lid up is leaving a free path for wealth to flow at speed away from your property – not to mention the fact that it isn't very nice to leave the toilet lid up in the first place.

So what do we want to encourage and what do we want to avoid or change?

Good Water/Negative Water

Natural water, fresh water, rainwater, clean water, slow-flowing water, water in front of your home and water that embraces your home are all types and examples of 'good' water, which you want to encourage into you life.

Old water, stagnant water, smelly acrid water, extremely fast-flowing water, water flowing directly to your door, water that flows behind your home or property, water that leaks, water that drips away and water that is contaminated, which completely overpowers your home or property, are all types of negative water. This is water that you could well do without, by draining away or by landscaping so that it works for you much more positively.

Get the flow flowing

The good water in our lives should be developed or encouraged. If you currently live in a property with a brook flowing through the garden, or with a pool, or by a lake, or are thinking of purchasing a property that has a natural water feature, just think of these considerations.

Is the water clean and either still or gently flowing? This water is ideal. The wealth is clean and flows gently into your life and moves slowly enough for you to be able to harness it if you so desire.

Is the water stagnant and dirty or pungent? This water is not good. It will reflect your own life; there will be no flow of wealth – in fact, there will be stagnation, which cannot generate any positive wealth. You can clean the water, but if this is not possible you may wish to consider filling in the pond or pool and then planting on the site. Water with no flow or life is very hard to clean and keep clean: you may be wasting your time and, as should be predicted, the mere presence of the water means you are wasting your money before you have even started to rectify the problem.

Does the water flow in front of the property? This is ideal, and if you can see the water coming and then it gently passes and flows away, you are in control of your wealth. If the water is fast-flowing and the source is hidden you won't know where the money comes from and it will be gone before you have had time to harness it or use it to your advantage. In cases like these you could landscape or place large rocks or boulders to move the flow path or slow it down. You could install a mirror or a window so that you can see the water moving towards you. To make huge changes like this it is wise to employ a consultant, discuss your concerns and come to a useful and practical conclusion.

If the water is leaking into a boggy part of the garden, get it fixed. It means your wealth is leaking and making your life boggy. If the pipes taking waste away from your property are not efficient or blocked, get them fixed. You do not wish to encourage effluent to linger around your home, and you don't want to build up stagnant, dirty fluid.

Is there is a slow drip or leak? Fix it before a bigger hole forms – it is much less expensive to solve a small problem than to deal with a replacement programme caused by leaving something untended and neglected. Do you start to see parallels with your own life and your own wealth? I hope so.

Finally, living by the sea or along a river is a very popular second-home or retirement option for many people. Installing a swimming pool in or by your own home could be a way to enjoy your home more. All these ideas involve large amounts of water. Remember how powerful large amounts of water can be and how if we get too much water all at once it can be devastating. Too much rainfall in one short space of time turns a river into a torrent bursting its banks. Turbulent weather, when the moon is affecting the seas and the weather is affecting the waves, can destroy coastlines and coastal dwellings. Pools constructed inside our homes or in our properties are expensive and time-consuming ... so you may want to consider buying a property with a great sea view, with the water flowing in front of your home at a distance, and you will get all the advantages with little of the problems. A home on the river would be better up on a hill rather than down by the river's edge. A swimming pool could be built outside of the house or in an outhouse so that it wouldn't quite overpower your home.

The water element is incredibly powerful, especially when Mother Nature takes control. The Water Detox is about harnessing and using that power to the best advantage. Read on.

ELECTROMAGNETIC FIELDS

If our bodies are 75 per cent water, and this is electrically charged, anything we come into contact with that has a strong charge itself will interfere with our own frequencies and the level at which we operate. This can be unsettling, disruptive and in some cases actually damaging.

We know that water is made up of hydrogen and oxygen. We also know that both hydrogen and oxygen have electrons associated with them. These are negatively charged, which put simply means that they spend all their time repelling each other, so that they are not able to stay together or near each other.

This means that water is very unstable, and that the slightest electrical or magnetic charge will have an effect on water. If we are mostly made of water then we are pretty unstable too – that is to say, we are very easily affected by any electrical or magnetic currents.

This effect can be very minor or it can be serious in that it interferes with the body's ability to operate on a healthy basis. In *Something in the Air*, Roger Coghill suggests that '... human beings are mostly made of water, anything we ingest will have a patterning effect, because all materials are slightly magnetic, even foods. When we are ill, we are suffering from improper patterning which is ultimately having a structural effect.' Working on the principle that everything has a magnetic charge, then everything can affect both our internal water and our electrical charges.

Coghill goes on to say: 'Even human beings are more sensitive to electric fields than previously believed. Because of its structure, water plays an important part in sensitivity, due to the movements of the hydrogen atoms ...'

This means that if we become exposed to regular amounts of electromagnetism we run the risk of changing the way our body is trying to work. Our body should work in harmony and any disruption of this will cause imbalance and eventually illness.

The influence of technology on our lives is incredibly liberating. We can get in touch with people via mobile phones wherever they are and wherever we are, we can microwave our food in a fraction of the time it takes to cook conventionally. Television brings us all the news and entertainment for a fun-packed evening and when we turn in for the night, we snuggle into our metal-framed bed in between sheets and a heated electric blanket. We are woken by a radio alarm chirping at our bedside, and we shower and then style our hair using dryers and heated curling tongs.

Life could hardly be more convenient, but all this convenience comes at a cost. The increases in electromagnetic fields, or EMFs, are to blame. We already have natural electromagnetic radiation from the sun, moon and earth, but some research shows that we are now bombarded with 150 million times more electromagnetic signals than our grandparents were. Many of these can be avoided, or we can take measures to protect ourselves against them.

You only need to drive under an electricity pylon and hear the radio frequency fuzz to experience the effect of an electromagnetic field. Turn the radio on near the hairdryer or curling tongs and you will get interference. Listen to a battery-operated radio, and hear the buzz when the washing machine does its spin cycle two floors away. All these are examples of electromagnetic radiation travelling through our day-to-day lives and our bodies.

But is this bad for our health or is it just yet another scare tactic?

Research suggests that it is bad and it is also the potential cause for many illnessess, diagnosed or otherwise. Roger Coghill's view is that our bodies have their own electrical frequencies involved in growth, repair, and cellular renewal – and that electric fields from machines and mobiles, microwaves and so on all have a detrimental effect on our own personal frequencies. His research finds that it is the alternating or 'AC' electric field part of the EMF that is dangerous to us, and that this is in action all the time an appliance is plugged in or fully charged.

It is suggested that illnesses such as ME, lethargy, headaches and some cancers are the result of our body's inability to repel electric fields. There are also groups that believe that EMFs disrupt our immune system's ability to cope.

There are many precautions you can take to reduce all unnecessary exposure to EMFs. Roger Coghill believes that we are resilient to short-term exposure, and should simply reduce their constant or longer-term presence in our lives. Even if final verdicts suggest that there is no real long-term danger or effect, we should still do all we can to reduce any potential interference.

We want positive and natural influences not negative and damaging ones.

Some reports say that long-term exposure is most likely to happen while you are sleeping in one spot for approximately 7 hours per day. It seems that sleeping next to a radio alarm can increase your exposure to EMFs at the very time your body needs to engage fully in its job of cell repair. General advice is to move the radio alarm so that it is at least 1.5 metres away from you. Alternatively, you can resort to the good old-fashioned wind-up alarm clock and get some real rest.

Electric blankets are reportedly tantamount to actually getting into an EMF, even when the blanket is turned off. You are still lying on a metallic grid and this will upset your own natural EMF. Ditch the blanket and just put on a warmer duvet or snuggle up closer to your partner.

Some reports allege that mobile phones could cause brain tumours. If you really need to use one, the best advice is to get an earpiece, which reduces the exposure of your head to the phone; or enclose the whole phone in a shield, available from mobile phone stores.

Unfortunately our parents were right all along – don't sit too close to the television. It seems that findings show this is good advice: we do tend to sit in front of the television for longer periods than is the case with any other household item, and advice suggests that we should sit no closer than 1.5 metres from the screen. Television screens emit 10 times the amount of electomagnetic radiation as computer screens do, so we should heed our parents just this once! Computer screens potentially give out negative ions so make sure you work at least 50 centimetres from the screen and take regular breaks.

There's not as much existing research on microwaves, but the common belief is that you shouldn't spend too much time close to one once it is turned on, and perhaps leave your food for a few minutes before tucking in. This is a useful piece of advice anyway, as microwaved food is generally too hot to eat immediately. You can check the security of your microwave by holding a radio near the door when it is turned on. If there is interference, there is likely to be leakage and repairs must be made or the appliance should be replaced.

We know we are affected all day long by varying currents, vibrations and resonance. Eliminating the potentially damaging ones or the ones that we don't know much about means we are truly detoxing our lives.

WATER SIGNS

As we have seen, there are many, many situations and scenarios where we are affected simply because we're mostly composed of water. Sorting out the water, and the forces affecting water, in and around us is a great way to enhance the Water Detox. Some of us have extra help in that we are born under an astrological water sign. This means that we have water in our life and our make-up from day one.

Looking at astrology, we can see that the 12 astrological signs are split into elements. Three are designated as water signs: Pisces, Cancer, and Scorpio. These signs are likely to feel the effects of water within them more than others are or at least be aware of differing feelings, while perhaps not putting them down to the water connection.

If you were not born under a water sign, you will still be affected as each astrological sign has an element of water within it.

Pisceans (20 February to 20 March)

The symbol for Pisces is two fish. Pisceans are creatures of change; they don't like to be doing the same thing for too long or be locked into one thing for too long. Pisceans are laid-back and go with the flow; you will rarely be able to whip them into a frenzy, but when you do you should beware. They are Neptune's people. They do not know greed and it is hard to get them to have an opinion on any extreme situation. Pisceans will often go for the easy way out and if they are disturbed, then all will be calm before nightfall. Pisceans, just like Scorpios and Cancerians, are to be found near water or will be drawn to water in some major aspect of their life. Water suits Pisceans – they thrive in it. They are, after all, fish disguised as humans!

Pisceans have a choice. Their sign shows fish facing in opposite directions, and they can swim any which way. They can travel to the surface and become successful and renowned, or they can swim to the bottom and become invisible and shady and even subjected to an alcoholic stupor. It is fair to say that a high percentage of alcoholics are Pisceans.

As fish, Pisceans must have water in their lives. If you are a Piscean and do not drink, swim or view water regularly, you should do so immediately and see how much you are freed and stimulated by this nourishing flow. The flower of the sign of Pisces is the water lily, which aptly depicts the nature and ability to survive with water and to flourish beautifully. Remove the water, and Pisceans dry up.

Cancerians (22 June to 23 July)

The symbol of the Cancerian is the crab, equally at home on land and in water. Unlike the Piscean, it can survive without water but needs it to fulfil 50 per cent of its being. Cancerians, like crabs, thrive in moonlight. Crabs come to land in the moonlight and it is this affinity with the planet that makes their moods changeable and strong. They match the tides, with their emotional pushing and pulling.

The term 'crabby' comes from the crab and Cancerians can be just that. They can snap and then hide in their hard shells until they are ready to come out. They always will, eventually, but you will feel the pinch of their claws if you question them when their emotions are moving in a watery way.

Spending time with these watery moon people will mean that you can catch their moods. Their affinity to water means their resonance and vibration is strong and will be passed on to you. Cancerians feed from water; they will go sailing or they will own boats or belong to a rowing club. To be on or in water is to be in the flow for Cancerians. Flow is also a huge part of their success: they can balance the flow of funds, of money, of income and outgoings. Cancerians tend to be wealthy people but they can be affected by moon madness. They are very interesting and deep people with many different aspects to their feminine moon side.

Scorpios (24 October to 22 November)

Scorpions are desert creatures, so they are about as far removed from water as you can get. But it is this contradiction that is perfect for Scorpios; you will never see the real emotion or the real reason behind a Scorpio. They hold the secrets to life's biggest questions and they can have and achieve just about anything they want to once they have put their minds to it. Living in the desert is no problem for this water sign.

Scorpios may live near the sea and they will empathise with the tides and the flow and depth of the sea. They will regard the water with great respect and be in no doubt as to its hidden depths and knowledge. The strong and silent qualities mirror the emotions of Scorpios.

Whatever you read on the face of a Scorpio, you should beware: absolutely anything could be going on behind those eyes and in that mind. Never cross a Scorpio because if you believe you have got away with anything you will feel the sharp sting in a day, month, or in many years, but sting it will. When the time is right the Scorpio will know and retaliate. Revenge is sweet for them, and they have an ocean of emotions and ideas to draw upon.

If you live with, associate, or work with any of these signs, you can watch and see how the changing phases of the moon affect them and how the weather can flip their mood. If you are one of these signs then check in with your emotions and moods and compare them with lunar phases. It may all start to make perfect sense. If you feel the moon's force, start to use it to your advantage. If you can do certain things in your life with the full strengthening support of the full moon, do so. If you need to discard or clear out, time it to follow the waning moon and you will achieve your goals much more readily.

WATER FOR HEALTH

We can work with water and we can add to our water. We've seen how we can work in line with our water to increase our strength and powers. We can also change the water we consume and actually increase its ability to heal. This is not just by filtration, but by adding something or, more specifically, the vibration of something.

If water has an electronic charge – and we know it does from the electron particles that are contained in the hydrogen and oxygen atoms it is made up of – then it has the ability to respond to other charges. Electronic pulses 'talk' to, and affect, each other every second of the day. You only have to place a mobile phone next to a land phone or television and you hear the two talking to each other by occasional beeps and interference. Radio callers are asked to turn off their radios as the interference makes the message change and difficult to hear clearly.

Everything has a charge or frequency, and if you put these together they will affect each other. If we change the vibration or frequency then we can change the effect. We can speed things up, or calm them down, and in turn they will have a speeding-up or a calming effect.

We can actually make water taste more refreshing or energising by simply stirring it vigorously or shaking it up before drinking it – try it if you don't believe me. Do an experiment with friends. Pour water into 3 glasses. Shake one, stir another, and leave the last as it is. Ask your friends which is the most refreshing. Give your water a vibe and see if it passes on.

The Memory of Water

Homeopathy is something I had been aware of for a long time. I had even taken homeopathic remedies and recommended them to clients and friends for the treatment of certain ailments. But it wasn't until I saw a play in London's West End, entitled *The Memory of Water*, that I began to realise the way homeopathic remedies worked and how their relationship with water was inextricable.

The word homeopathy derives from the Greek word *homoios*, meaning 'like', and the word *patheis*, meaning 'suffering'. This word was used because it was based in the belief that like cures like – an understanding from as far back as the days of the renowned Greek physician Hippocrates. The belief, put simply, is that administering minute amounts of the substance that actually causes the same symptoms or problems can bring about the cure of the illness or the disease.

Homeopathy as we know it today was founded by a man named Samuel Hahnemann in Germany in the 1790s. Hahnemann first published his findings in a paper, *The Law of Similars*, in 1796. He had found that by giving people small doses of something that caused the same side effects as the illness they actually had, they recovered speedily. For instance, taking quinine gave him all the symptoms of a person suffering from malaria. Giving small doses to someone actually suffering from malaria was found to cure them.

In order to get the correct amounts or dosage, Hahnemann developed a technique he called 'potentising'. He would dilute the substances with water and alcohol, and subject them to rigorous shaking – a process he termed 'succussion'. This dilution and shaking would allow him to prescribe even the deadliest of substances quite safely, and with very good effects and cures.

The process of succussion was stumbled upon by accident. It seems that he was using his remedies for treating his patients with some success. However, the patients who he travelled to would recover much more rapidly, and Hahnemann realised that the shaking of the bottles during the horseback or carriage ride to his patients' homes was doing the trick! He therefore introduced the process of succussion to every one of his potentised remedies.

The principle is that a minute amount of something is big enough to cause an effect within the body and rally the immune system, but not so much that the immune system is overtaken. In doing this, the body's immunity becomes successful in recognising the illness and finding a cure.

This minuscule amount could almost be termed a 'non' amount. The original substance is introduced to the water and succussion takes place. This leaves what is called an imprint of the original substance on the pure water. That is to say, the water 'remembers' the structure of the organism or mineral or plant extract that was shaken in it. This water is then diluted so much that there really is none of the original substance detectable – just the memory of it having once been there.

Hahnemann developed three rules that he established as the principles of homeopathy:

- A substance that causes a set of symptoms in a healthy body can also be expected to cure the same symptoms in a sick body.

- Potentising or 'diluting' a substance increases its efficacy without endangering the patient.

- Homeopathy is holistic and treats the whole body, not only the symptoms of the illness.

So there truly is nothing left of the original substance – just the memory, template, resonance, vibration or energy of it. This will work on the body's memory, template, resonance, vibration and energy. The whole body is affected. It's a truly holistic treatment.

Homeopathic remedies should be looked after carefully. As they consist of the memory of a vibration or the energy of a substance, you should not subject the remedy to anything other than the energy of the patient it is going to treat.

I personally take homeopathic remedies while flying, along with flower remedies (see page 174). I found that at one point in my life my fear was getting to the stage that I would choose not to travel if I could possibly avoid it, and if I couldn't avoid it I would then become very tense, especially if flying without my partner. I was prescribed the remedies and was reminded not to allow them through the X-ray security arch we are all asked to walk through at airports. This makes perfect sense, as the radiation will simply realign the vibration of the water and 'wipe' the memory, rendering the remedy useless. (There is one point, though, worth considering. If you do see someone taking remedies that they have passed through the X-ray please do not be helpful and go up to them to tell them that they have made them useless. If they need them to work then hopefully they may work on the placebo level if not on the treatment level. If someone told me that I had ruined my remedies before boarding then I really don't know how I would get on the plane!)

If you visit a homeopath, you need to give them a lengthy history of your health and your life. A homeopath will not have a certain remedy for a certain illness but will take into account many factors about yourself and your lifestyle before prescribing remedies. They will also change levels over the period of prescription, as different amounts work for different people. Establishing this amount can take time. Also, you should expect the cure to follow the rule of 12, just as a lot of Chinese medicine does. This means that for 12 months you have had the problem, you will undergo the treatment for 1 month. If you have had irritable bowel syndrome for 3 years, expect to take remedies for at least 3 months. If you are taking homeopathy to prevent or to pro act to a condition, the response will be more immediate. I take homeopathic remedies if I am expecting a visit to the dentist or a visit to the hospital in order to prevent any bruising or scarring, and to speed up the healing process. I also take homeopathic remedies on holiday to stop the mosquitoes from dining out on my blood for two weeks . . .

You should also remember not to drink caffeine or use peppermint toothpaste while you are taking remedies or while they are in your stomach, as both these substances will cancel out the efficacy of the pill. Your homeopath should be able to give you herbal toothpaste and caffeine (but you shouldn't be drinking it on a detox programme anyway!).

FLOWER REMEDIES

Extracts from flowers and plants are some of the oldest forms of medicine that we know today. Indeed, some of the most potent drugs that we are aware of are plant extracts. Heroin is derived from the poppy, and digitalis from the beautiful foxglove.

All these medicines use the plant's bark or leaves, but not many of them use the actual flower itself.

Flower remedies use the flowerhead, as this is thought to be the ultimate manifestation of the power and beauty of the individual plants. The bloom or the blossom will have the best curative effect. Flower essences work more on the energy, the emotions and spirit, than the body. We all know exactly how uplifting and exhilarating it can be to walk into a beautiful garden in flower or to see a room full of beautiful fresh-cut flowers, or indeed to open the door to someone carrying a bunch of flowers intended for us. Well, think of that feeling and then bottle it. This will go some way towards explaining the reason for flower remedies.

Typically, we need to look to ancient tribes. These people lived off the land and used vegetation – the first and earliest indications that flowers were used for healing. Australian aboriginals once drank the dew on fresh flower blooms; Native Americans would take flowers and sit among them, or walk in the early morning dew to absorb the full effect of the flowers. Kahuna Indians of Hawaii wore garlands of flowers to celebrate the earth.

As history has a habit of repeating itself, some of the most popular flower remedies are those from Australia, made from native Australian bush plants and flowers. But Edward Bach's are probably the most famous.

Bach developed a system of remedies using the flowers from wild plants, trees and bushes. He placed the flowers in bowls of pure water and then left these bowls outside in the sunlight. In doing so he believed that the life force or the vibration of these beautiful wild flowers would pass to the water and then the water could be used to take as a medicine.

Bach was a homeopath, a bacteriologist and a pathologist, and it was his understanding of homeopathy and its effectiveness linked to his love of wild flowers and the calming influence that they had on him that led him to develop the Bach Flower Remedies.

Unlike Hahnemann, who introduced homeopathy to cure illness holistically, Bach intended his remedies to work on specific emotions. He believed that the emotions and the personality were the route to full health. A positive mind would ultimately lead to a healthy body. But like Hahnemann, he totally believed in the memory of the water as a therapeutic and curative force.

There are 38 Bach Remedies in the original groupings, and these are separated into 7 subsets:

- **Fear** Rock Rose, Mimulus, Cherry Plum, Aspen and Red Chestnut.

- **Uncertainty** Cerato, Scleranthus, Gentian, Gorse, Hornbeam and Wild Oat.

- **Apathy or insufficient interest in present circumstances** Clematis, Honeysuckle, Wild Rose, Olive, White Chestnut, Mustard and Chestnut Bud.

- **Loneliness** Water Violet, Impatiens and Heather.

- **Oversensitivity to influence and ideas** Agromony, Centaury, Walnut and Holly.

- **Despondency and despair** Larch, Pine, Elm, Sweet Chestnut, Star of Bethlehem, Willow, Oak and Crab Apple.

- **Overcare or welfare of others** Chicory, Vervain, Vine, Beech and Rock Water.

These remedies can be taken on their own or they can be combined to make the remedy more specific to your own personal emotion or concern. The remedies are sold in small bottles and the water dilution is preserved in brandy. You can get Bach Remedies from many high street chemists and health food shops. They are great for self-diagnosis and administration. The same rules apply as for homeopathy. Do not subject them to radioactive, X-ray or magnetic influences or you will find that the water is reprogrammed and the remedies rendered ineffective.

You can make your own flower remedies and use these at home for yourself or actually in your home to lift the spirits of the place where you live.

Just as Bach did, you can choose your flower and place it in a bowl of clear, pure, fresh water. Make sure that you pick the flower early in the morning, when dew is still on the petals, and that there are no pollutants like pesticides or insecticides on the flowers. An organic garden is perfect for taking flowers to make your own remedies. Take a clean bowl and fill with natural water – spring or natural mineral water is preferable. Place it in bright sun and put the flower or flowers in it. Leave for several hours. Once the water has received the vibration of the flowers for a suitable length of time you can use the water just as it is. Use it to spray a room or wash your clothes, or use as a body splash or to rinse your head and hair. Alternatively, if you want to keep the essence and make it last, mix an equal amount of it with brandy. This will ensure that nothing goes off, and make the tincture safe to take internally for a period of time.

You should endeavour to use these essences when they are quite fresh. You can simply make more as and when you need them. There is also a strong feeling that your remedies should follow the seasons. Make essences in the summer with the full summer blooms and make them in the winter with the wonderful rich petals from winter-flowering bushes and plants. Nature has reasons for growing different plants at different times, and to benefit from these seasonal supports is quite a wonderful way to stay 'in tune' with your surroundings.

CRYSTAL ESSENCES OR SPRITZES

Flower essences and homeopathic medicines are not the only things that we can use to help improve the health and quality of our lives. It is possible to make remedies out of almost anything if you understand and subscribe to the 'memory of water' theory.

If the water that you place an object or plant into takes on the resonance and vibration of that plant or object, then essences know no bounds.

Essences made using crystals, gems and precious metals work in exactly the same way. Crystal healing is very old. Stones, gems and crystals all come from the earth, where they form over millions of years, and have their own powerful healing and regenerative properties. They are natural, organic objects. Obviously you cannot take them internally unless they are totally edible and digestible. In certain cases they can be ground down and taken as a powder. Indeed, gold and silver are very precious metals that are used quite frequently in Western medicine.

Crystal and gem therapy has been used for centuries to heal the spiritual and energetic harmony within the body. Crystal energy is particularly good when working with the resonance of the energy channels within the body – the chakras, the meridians and the auric field. If you work with homeopathic, flower and gem remedies, you will certainly be addressing your needs for mind, body and spirit.

Just like flowers, each and every gem or crystal, precious or semi-precious, also has a healing property. Crystals have been used for adornment, protection and healing. If we could hear them talk they would have amazing stories to tell and tremendous wisdom and knowledge.

Traditionally, we can benefit from these properties by holding or wearing a crystal, or having a treatment with the physical crystal present. Crystal healing works on the premise that every crystal vibrates on a different but constant frequency. Selecting a crystal or gem that resonates or vibrates at the beneficial rate for the patient will ultimately bring the body into balance and harmony.

When considering making your own remedies, you should look into the crystals that you are drawn to or ones that you have heard of. It is often said that the crystals or even flowers that you are attracted to are the ones that have the properties you need to create total balance or to feel 'complete'. In the same way, we find our friends and partners for life. We are usually drawn to people who complement us or who we feel nourished by or feel good with.

Many people who don't practise crystal therapy do consider it normal practice to have diamonds in their engagement rings. They probably just thought it was because diamonds were expensive, and so denote commitment! Take a look at what the diamond signifies, and see that you could even benefit from diamond crystal essence.

There is a crystal for every situation and every emotion. Detoxing comes with using them for cleansing and clearing in fact. Look at some of the more common crystals in the table below, and see how we can include them in our life, how they can boost and enhance – and how they can make us balanced and harmonious. See page 181 for how to make the crystal elixir or essence.

Crystal	Benefits
Diamond	We take it for granted that engagement rings usually include a diamond. The diamond signifies loyalty, fidelity and the bond between man and woman. Diamond is pure, strong, durable – completely appropriate in a piece of jewellery used as a prelude to the marriage ceremony. If you want to be steadfast, or loyal, or to feel commitment, you could try to make an elixir from any diamond jewellery you have and feel the effects.
Amber	Amber brings wisdom and balance, and holds secrets of the earth. Amber is healing. It can banish negative thoughts and energy. It is also a kidney tonic.
Tiger's eye	Tiger's eye is for protection and can help you draw on your own resources without draining you. It can balance your digestion. It helps develop your own intuition and is reported to give great confidence.
Opal	The opal cleanses the blood and kidneys and keeps insulin levels balanced. It encourages spontaneity and creativity but keeps you emotionally stable. Opals are good for passion.
Quartz	One of the more common stones, quartz is probably also one of the most powerful. It is used to cleanse and

revitalise. It can be used to dissipate bad energy and regulate good energy. Often used near computer screens to prevent harmful rays and static, it is also great for stimulating immunity.

Rose quartz
Rose quartz is a stone of love. Its pinkish hue is romantic and healing. It helps self-love as well as love for others, and works on the heart emotionally and physically. It encourages circulation and blood flow and brings about healing.

Fluorites (all types)
Fluorites come in many forms: they are a big family. Fluorites protect. They are grounding and centring. They help release toxins and help with cell growth and muscle damage. They can also boost creativity and sexuality.

Agate
Agates are calming and cooling, grounding and harmonising. They boost our confidence and equip us with the ability to move on. Blue agate brings about balance and strengthens bones by speeding up the healing process.

Labradorite
This oddly named crystal is fabulous for aiding digestion and metabolism. It protects and recharges and enables our own intuition and insight to grow. It is also the duty of labradorite to recharge all other stones on the planet. It cancels negative energy and promotes positive energy.

Emerald
Emeralds are grounding and balancing, physically and emotionally. They are calming and restful. Emeralds can enhance muscle healing and promote heart health. Emeralds will never let you forget – they are the stones of memory.

Lapis lazuli
Lapis is good for stress. It balances and harmonises on a mind, body and spirit level. It promotes immunity and cleansing, creativity and objectivity. It is an all-round balancer.

Citrine
Citrine is less common but just as valuable. It is balancing and cleansing. It works on the digestive system and the circulation, and enhances creativity and encourages motivation.

Tourmaline
This stone is very cleansing, great for detoxification. It purifies and boosts immunity and is very rejuvenating. It is also very balancing and grounding, as are many of the green gemstones.

Malachite
This is another fabulous green stone with amazing properties. It is 'the stone of transformation', according to the British Fossil Association. It can help in times of great or small change, and allows you to move forward and relinquish the past.

Sodalite
Great for elimination, sodalite boosts the kidneys and liver. It aids the metabolism and immune system. It is calming and balancing.

Amethyst
Amethyst, from the quatz family, is a great all-rounder. It heals and protects, helps the kidneys and liver, boosts circulation, balances the nervous system, aids immunity and digestion, and promotes heart health. It is used in meditation and visualisation and can often be found as a large crystal emanating energy and warmth.

Snowflake obsidian (Apache tears)
These stones encourage self-love and banish self-doubt. They keep balance through times of change and allow you to move forwards, letting go of past fears or memories. They are very positive stones that keep you in control when you most need to be. Snowflake obsidian also helps to heal skin.

Turquoise
Like Apache tears, turquoise is a stone often worn by Native Americans. Most helpful with healing and protection, it promotes self-worth and self-realisation, and is supportive through change. Turquoise banishes negativity and promotes positive feelings of health and wealth. Turquoise is an all-round healer of the whole body, mind and spirit.

This is only a minute selection of the most common stones, gems and crystals that we can use in crystal therapy, but it may just be enough to show you how they can support and enhance our lives.

How to Make a Crystal Essence

To make a crystal or gem essence elixir, or spritz, follow exactly the same steps as you would to make a flower essence. Take a clean bowl and fill with water – spring or natural mineral water is preferable. Place it in bright sunlight, put the crystal in it and leave for several hours. Once the water has received the vibration for a suitable length of time, you can use it just as it is, take it in small amounts or drops on the tongue, use it to spray a room to space clear, or bathe in it. If you want to keep the essence and make it last, you should mix it with an equal amount of brandy. This will ensure that nothing goes off and make the tincture safe to take for a period of time. You must make sure that the crystal is very clean and that nothing falls off the crystal into the water for you to swallow.

You can of course buy crystal remedies to use, but it's not nearly so much fun.

ANIMAL ESSENCES

Something else that is relatively new to the market but totally fascinating and leads as a natural extension to the Native American belief in the power of animals is animal essences.

Now before you imagine parts of animal being left out in the sun in a bowl of water for several hours, or get a mental picture of trying to hold your very well-trained Alsatian in the bath on a sunny day ... you have to remember we are talking vibration or energy, not the actual animal. Animal essences were introduced before you needed to visualise or imagine the animal and its qualities to take the medicine. Now you can actually take the medicine internally with these products.

Reading the literature on them, we are assured that 'animal essences, like flower and gem elixirs, are "vibrational remedies" – each of the essences contains the vibrational imprint and energy of the animal but does not contain any animal part'.

So you can breathe easy. They are totally vegetarian. The essences are actually made during a ceremonial process of attunement in the wild. This process includes the invocation of the spirit of the animal, and meditation and attunement with the animal involved. The essence simply contains the vibrational imprint and energy of the animal.

The essences respect the water's ability to hold this imprint, to hold it in mind, and to give us the full value of the great properties of some of the most amazing creatures on this earth. Animals have always been significant for native peoples. Animals represent power, wisdom, strength and guidance.

The Native American tribes use animals as their totems or gods to pray to and consult for spiritual guidance. Animals represent different characteristics and strengths and the Native Americans use this symbolism to guide their lives. We can use some of this symbolism to help in guiding ourselves to get where we want to be in our lives.

Animals have their own life force. We know that spending time with animals can benefit therapeutically. Animals are used in hospitals and homes to relax and inspire patients or residents, and in therapy because they are guileless and interact with us honestly. Their energy is comforting and calming: think of the soothing presence of a cat on your lap when you are stressed. If you couple this with their individual characteristics, you will have different types of spirit and/or energy. This is the essence of animal medicine. You can find out about yourself through the animal energy that visits you or that you think about or summon into your life. Listen to what they are telling you and act accordingly. Remember, animals don't tell lies and have no hidden agendas; they just tell the truth.

This medicine can be used for inspiration, confidence, support and guidance. It can help you through the more difficult challenges you face. It can also be lighthearted, enabling you to be lighthearted and frivolous.

Indeed this medicine can be taken for everything. You can choose what you take and when you take it, and you can use it just whenever you want to. It's a wonderful tool to add to our personal medicine chest. It visits when least expected and can be called upon as and when you need it. And you don't even need to use the essences. You are probably already using animal medicine in one way or another – or at least, it is probably already in your life without you knowing it.

I've sketched in why animals have much to offer us therapeutically. Now let's take a closer look at precisely why they have this power. See the table opposite detailing the specific qualities each animal can impart to us.

Wild animals live on this earth quite freely, and have evolved many ways to survive. When we domesticate them for our own pleasure and use, they lose some of their independence but none of their 'animal instincts'. Pet cats will still bring in shrews, mice and birds despite having a bowlful of food served to them on a regular basis. Horses at the riding stables will still shy away if you approach their blind spot, or kick out.

Every animal has a certain set of qualities. Every animal can help in totally different ways. I have picked a few of the more common animals to start with, but every animal has medicine.

If you aren't using the essences, you can use your imagination to invoke the animal's power. The beauty of animal medicine is that it can happen anywhere, any time. In a meeting, if your job description is being discussed or there is a period of change facing your company, just imagine the crow on a perch behind you, sharing your situation. Crows see universal law and justice and crows see and help with change. Bring in the crow, and see change happen for the better.

Coyote medicine is my favourite. When I get a little too serious or bogged down by deadlines or get nervous about demonstrations or public speaking, I just stroke my pet coyote that hangs out by my right leg. He will often wander away, but just when I need the support, like a faithful but lighthearted dog he comes straight back to heel, looking after me. With coyote medicine I can balance just about anything. Now I can also take the essence itself.

Other people can take this medicine either by visualisation or as an actual essence, and you can send this medicine to others. If you have children at college and it is exam time, or if your friends are travelling the world and you are worried about them, think of an animal and send them the medicine or have it mailed directly from the distributors. In the same way, if an animal visits you, if you open your curtains one morning and there are birds on your lawn, look up their medicine and see what the day holds. You can then increase this by taking the essence as before. If you are out walking and a horse rides by, what are you being told, what is being sent to help you? When sitting in a traffic jam and you see a mouse in the corner of the alleyway, are you looking at the details or are you getting bogged down in the detail and not seeing the wood for the trees? What essence are you being told to try?

Animal	Medicine
Swan	Beauty and grace. Power from within.
Spider	New creations and creating new experiences.
Horse	Ability to travel and find freedom. Your own personal power.
Ant	Hard work will give you rewards.
Wolf	Guarding and protecting. Loyalty.
Owl	Truth and vision.
Dolphin	Breath and life. Joy.
Bat	Facing your fear, seeing through everything to get to the truth.
Deer	Caring, compassion, gentleness.
Bear	Power, physical and inner strength.
Dog	Loyalty.
Squirrel	Preparation, being industrious and prepared for any eventuality.
Coyote	Having fun, lightening up, not being so serious.
Whale	Creativity.
Eagle	Getting things in perspective, taking the bigger view to sort things out.

Snake	Change, rebirth, wisdom. Magic and enchantment.
Butterfly	Transformation and change.
Fox	Cunning. Imagination and interpretation.
Crow	Magic and change. Secrecy. Justice.
Cat	Independence and mystery.

So use the essences or your imaginative power – whichever, you will find that animal medicine is so versatile and so much fun. You can be just whoever you want to be and you can do whatever takes your fancy or whatever you need to do when you use it. Animal medicine is empowering and will keep you young. Animals do not work with your age, they work with your being.

WATER VIBRATION FOR RELAXATION

Everything in the world has a vibration or resonance of its own, whether it be animal, vegetable or mineral. Our resonant frequency reacts with our water and electrical pulses. If something has a similar resonant frequency we are affected, and if someone or something has an opposing resonant frequency we are also affected. If you have ever heard an opera singer or choir hit a high note and been reduced to tears, then it is the frequency that has hit your nerve. Ella Fitzgerald, the vocalist, famously smashes glasses by mimicking their resonant frequency, which is extremely high. The sound shakes the frequency of the glass to the extent that it explodes.

Both colour and music have resonant frequencies of their own. These will be high, low or medium. High frequency will invigorate and enliven while low frequency will relax and calm. You can actually see these vibrations by placing a glass of water on top of a speaker while playing music. Try different types of music and see how the vibrations differ. This effect also occurs within our bodies – our own water is moved and affected in the same way.

Colour also has a frequency: red is one of the strongest and green and blue are two of the softest. The colour surrounding us has a similar effect to the music. It will resonate with the water content of our bodies and relax or invigorate, depending on our own personal frequency.

When we are stressed we should look to ways in which water can help settle the mind or the churning stomach; ways that we can calm ourselves and get our bodies and emotions back into balance and flow. If we block our feelings or we become too tense, we cannot operate efficiently on any level. The Water Detox is about opening up and being able to deal with situations in a calm way. Holding on to unwanted emotions or thoughts is definitely 'tox'.

Have you ever found yourself using these phrases?

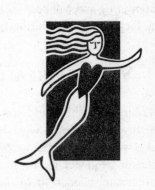

- 'Getting with the vibe'
- 'Getting back into the flow'
- 'In the swim'
- 'Waves of emotion'
- 'Washed over me'
- 'Drowning in stress/sadness'
- 'Dip your toe'
- 'I feel it in my waters'
- 'Totally immersed in . . .'

These are all phrases we use when talking about the feelings of being stressed or out of control, recovering from a stressful period or trying something new as a way of recovering. They all have watery or vibration connections, they all refer to our internal flow being out of balance, disrupted or stagnant. We talk of experimentation being like trying out new waters, for instance.

It's as if we know it is in fact our 'water' that is out of balance.

Well, if our own water content can be affected or rebalanced by changing or affecting its vibration, flow or resonance, then we should consider ways to do this so that we have our own in-built stress reduction and relaxation tools.

Try some of these techniques when things are getting a bit too much and turn a turmoiled or raging sea into calm waters.

Colour Healing

The use of colours in healing is nothing new. The use of colours in our life is nothing new either. Most of us are very aware of how colour affects mood. Next time you look at colour, ask yourself, 'How does it make me feel?' Every colour has a frequency and a vibration. Some are exhilarating and some are relaxing. 'Like a red rag to a bull', 'The tranquil turquoise sea', 'sunshine yellow' – these phrases refer to a mood or quality of colour rather than the look of the colour. When we do yoga or meditation we are asked to visualise colours. This indicates deeper states of relaxation and release. Colour is not just pretty to look at; its vibration can truly change our state of mind and emotion. Get the water in your body to resonate peace and tranquillity.

Colour	Qualities
Red	Red is a stimulating colour with a high frequency. In Chinese medicine it denotes fire and energy. It is associated with the liver and the clearing of toxins – so it's great for detoxification. It is supposed to enhance circulation and signify strength, life force and vitality.
Yellow	Yellow is a very grounding colour; it stimulates mental clarity and thoughtfulness. Yellow is associated with the lymph flow and the intestines, and is very good for processing in any detoxification programme. The frequency is fairly high but not as high as red.
Green	Green is a relaxing colour; it is often used in relaxation rooms. The green room in the theatre is used to relax and calm. Green is about balance of the body and brain. Green is a wood element colour in Chinese medicine. It is about growth and development and it is also the colour for detoxification via the liver and kidneys. Green is low frequency, relaxing and hypnotic.

Purple   Purple is also relaxing, but in a meditative way – it takes us to a spiritual state. It calms the kidneys and the adrenal glands. It is also the colour used to calm high blood pressure and to encourage sleep. Purple is one of the 'highest' colours in Indian medicine. The crown energy at the top of our head is often depicted as purple, denoting connection with spirit. Purple has low resonance and vibration.

Orange   Orange stimulates the lungs, and is a decongestant colour. It clears the way for the life force and it represents life and energy. Many Eastern religious orders wear orange. Orange has a higher vibration than purple.

Blue   Blue is cooling and calming. It is the colour for communication, for saying what you mean in a cool and considered way. Blue is the colour to reduce inflammations, physically or emotionally, and it is the colour of water, cooling and calming and refreshing. Blue has a lower resonance for relaxation.

White   White is low frequency; it is about peace and calm. People who have a near-death experience talk about a calming white light. White is about comfort and also truth. White is a colour that reduces or removes pain.

The next time you feel stressed or annoyed see if colour healing can bring you back into frequency. You don't need to redecorate each time you wish to change your mood, but think in terms of surroundings and also colour.

- Red: wear something red to stimulate the senses and increase the flow.

- Yellow: go out in the sunshine (with sun protection of course) and bathe in the yellow light.

- Green: go for a calming and grounding walk in the woods or sit on a green lawn and look around you at the amazing array of green colours and plants.

- Purple: buy purple bed sheets or purple cushions for deep sleep and stress reduction.

- Orange: wear orange to bring life and vitality, or buy orange flowers to enliven yourself and a room.

- Blue: walk by a river or sea shore. Take a bath with relaxing blue bubbles.

Use colour to balance your flow.

Get with the Vibe

Music, of course, has a vibration and frequency. We can see this by simply placing a hand on top of a speaker while the music is on. The vibration resonates through the body.

Lullabies relax and send babies off to sleep. Massage and complementary therapy treatments are nearly always accompanied by the sounds of gentle waters, classical music, dolphin calls, or Pan pipes. All these sounds are resonating at a deep relaxation level.

Nightclubs whip people into a frenzy with the heavy repetitive beat. Dancers can change mood simply by hearing the music; no drugs or alcohol are necessary to change the state.

Whatever the kind of music we are talking about, it all has the ability to change moods, to relax, to invigorate, to energise and to calm. Next time you feel in a mood or emotionally upset, or if you just want to wake up before you go out for the evening, choose your music carefully, get the beat you want and feel the sounds wash over you.

Feel the Force

Just as earth's water is affected by the gravitational or magnetic pull of the planets, so we are affected by that same gravitational or magnetic pull. If we are in balance then our body's waters are balanced and in free flow, with no blockages or stagnation. If we are out of balance we have stagnation and build-up of fluid.

We can magnetise our own water to get it back into balance, either by magnetising the water we drink or placing magnets directly on the areas of inbalance or pain. This will have an effect on the electrons inside our bodies and the electrons surrounding every atom of water either inside or outside our bodies.

If you take yourself back to school science lessons, you may remember the time you were asked to place a magnet in among some iron filings. As soon as the magnet is in place, the once randomly scattered filings form into a natural arc around the field of the magnet. If you placed two magnets facing each other, the patterns become more intricate but just as balanced.

It is this balancing effect that we want to benefit from.

To magnetise water, you need to pour it into the glass or jug and then stand it on the magnet for at least 8 hours. This will improve and balance the vibration and gravitational pull of the water atoms and in turn this is reported to have the same effects on your body.

To magnetise yourself directly you simply place a small magnet on the area of pain or discomfort. If you know about reflex points in the feet you can place the magnet on the relevant meridian point and if you have done work with chakras you can place the magnet on the chakra in need of work.

You can buy magnets for medicinal use from a company called Magnet Therapy Ltd and find a practitioner from the British Biomagnetic Association (see page 197). There is also some suggested further reading on this vast subject (see page 194).

SOME FINAL THOUGHTS …

There is something else to consider: how old is the water we drink, and where does it come from? Think about where it has been before and consider the route it took to get to you, to the glass in front of you or to the bath you just ran. We get our water from bottles or from the tap and we don't give it a second thought. How does it get to the bottle or tap and where was it before then?

- You could be drinking water that has been drunk by soldiers in ancient Rome.

- You could be bathing in water that has had a starring role in Niagara Falls.

- Your glass of water could have rained on a royal wedding.

- Your glass of water could have been part of a tragic avalanche.

- Millions of people could have tasted your water before you.

- This could be the first time that the water you hold in your glass has ever been tasted by a human being.

- Your water could have had previous employment as a cloud, a river, a stream, a lake, a waterfall, a sweaty run, a swim with dolphins, a Roman bath, a mud pool, an icicle, a snowstorm, a torrential downpour, or the morning dew.

- Your water could have been part of a London fog or the blizzard around the summit of Mount Everest.

- It might have steamed away a common cold or relaxed a rugby team in the sauna.

- It may have washed away the troubles of the day, or it could have been used to baptise a new baby.

- It may have been part of a Mississippi River flood, or have propelled a speedboat into Monaco . . .

However and whatever water is used for, that glass of fresh, clean water directly in front of you could have been around since the dawn of time. Water is cyclical, it is used, it gets poured away, it goes into processing plants, it can be used to water plants, it will evaporate into the atmosphere and it can then fall as rain on a reservoir for someone else to drink or into the sea to swim in . . . the possibilities are endless, and amazing.

There is nothing new in water. What is new is our outlook and our knowledge of just how crucial it is to our total health and vitality.

Instruction Manual: Dry Skin Brushing

Dry skin brushing is quite simple to do, extremely effective – and nothing comes near it for waking you up in the morning. Now that you have plenty of excellent reasons to dry skin brush, the next step is to know how to do it effectively.

1. Find a natural bristle brush, a loofah, a dry flannel or a mitt. The bristles or flannel, etc., should be firm but not hard. You will be brushing your skin quite vigorously all over your body – the skin on your stomach is softer than the skin on your shins or forearms. Do not wet or moisturise the skin, as this may cause dragging.

2. Having undressed to your underwear, or preferably with no clothes on, stand or sit in a position that enables access to all parts of the body. The edge of the bed with feet on pillows is quite good, or sitting on the edge of the bath with one foot up on the toilet seat works well.

3. Start at the feet and systematically work up towards the top of your body. All strokes should be towards the heart – the heart is a wonderful pump for pumping the blood down throughout the body, but both blood and lymph need extra help to work against gravity and return through the system; if we brush away from the heart it may cause faintness or disrupt the normal flow.

   Each stroke should be long and firm. Place the brush/mitt on the ankle and firmly brush up to the knee; repeat several times until you have covered the entire calf and shin several times. When you have completed the lower leg then move up to the knee. The next strokes should run from the knee to the top of the thigh and over the buttocks.

4. Brush both arms, from the wrist to the shoulder. The neck and shoulder area should be treated more gently, as the flesh here is very delicate. Work from the top of the arm, up and over the shoulder and gently up the neck to the base of the skull.

5. When brushing the stomach, use gentle circular strokes in a clockwise direction. This will follow the flow in your intestines and will not disrupt any bowel functions.

6. You must only brush the face with a soft facial brush or flannel, as the skin here is very delicate and can be damaged if the brush is too hard.

The whole process should only take 3 or 4 minutes, and you should feel quite invigorated when you have finished. Your skin will tingle and you will feel warm as you have stimulated and increased your circulation. You will soon notice quite a difference in your skin: it feels smoother with a softer texture, and the dry patches will have all disappeared. Just spend a little time each day on this exercise and you will be pleasantly surprised at the dramatic results.

Further Reading

Your Body's Many Cries for Water, Dr Fereydoon Batmanghelidj, Worthing: The Therapist Ltd, 1997.

Something in the Air, Roger Coghill (available from: Coghill Research Laboratories, Lower Race, Pontypool, Gwent NP4 5UH).

Water – Pure Therapy, Alice Kavounas, London: Kyle Cathie Ltd, 2000.

H_2O: Healing Water for Mind and Body, Anna Selby, London: Collins & Brown, 2000.

H_2O: The Beauty and Mystery of Water, Hans Silvester, Bernard Fischesser and Marie-France Dupuis-Tate, London: Thames & Hudson, 2000.

The Healing Energies of Water, Charlie Ryrie, London, Gaia Books, 1999.

Water Feng Shui for Wealth, Lillian Too, Konsep Books, 1998.

Dolphin Healing, Horace Dobbs, London: Piatkus Books, 2000.

Raphael's Astronomical Ephemeris of the Planets

This little booklet tells you the movement of every planet throughout the year. Apart from being intriguing left lying on your coffee table, it is also a great way to find the moon's exact state for every day of the year. These books are published annually and are in the astronomy section of the bookshop or can be ordered through Macmillan Distribution on 01256 302699.

Vibrational Medicine for the 21st Century, Richard Gerber, London: Piatkus Books, 2000.

Look at the following websites for further information on a number of issues I've covered:

www.bottledwater.org
www.animalessences.com
www.alaskanessences.com

Useful Addresses and Contacts

These addresses are useful for finding what you might need on your Water Detox programme.

Practitioners in Colonics
Colonic International Association
16 Englands Lane
London NW3 4TG
020 7483 1595

Feng Shui Courses and Information
The School of Feng Shui
Hands Farm, Middlefield Lane
Newbold-on-Stour
Warwickshire CV37 8TX
01789 459288
info@fengshui-school.co.uk
www.fengshui-school.co.uk

Bach Flower Remedies
The Edward Bach Centre
Mount Vernon
Bakers Lane
Sotwell
Oxon OX10 0PZ
01491 834678

International Flower Essence Repertoire
The Living Tree
Milland
Near Liphook
Hants GU30 7JS

Aromatherapy Blends
Aromatherapy Associates Ltd
6 Great West Trading Estate
Brentford
Middlesex TW8 9DN
020 8569 7030

Essential Oils
Call for full brochure:
- **Fragrant Earth**
  01458 831216

International Dolphin Watch
10 Melton Road
North Ferriby
East Yorkshire HU14 3ET
01482 645789
www.IDW.org

Magnetic Therapy Ltd
Freepost (MR9954)
Ellesmere Centre
Walkden-Worsley
Manchester M29 9DU
www.magnetictherapy.co.uk

For Magnet Therapy Practitioners
British Biomagnetic Association
The Williams Clinic
31 Marychurch Road
Torquay
Devon TQ1 3JF

For Water Sports

The British Sub-Aqua Club (BSAC)
Telford's Quay
South Pier Road
Ellesmere Port
Cheshire CH65 4FL
0151 350 6200
www.BSAC.com

British Canoe Union
Adbolton Lane
West Bridgford
Nottingham NG2 5AS
0115 9821100
www.bcu.org.uk

The Ski Club of Great Britain
The White House
57–63 Church Road
Wimbledon
London SW19 5SB
020 8410 2000
www.skiclub.co.uk

Royal Yachting Association
RYA House
Ensign Way
Hamble
Southampton SO31 4YA
0845 345 0400
www.rya.org.uk

Index

aches and pains 145–6
acidity 139–40, 145
agate 179
ageing, premature 129–30
alarm clocks 166
alcoholic drinks
  consuming water with 22
  diuretic effects of 44, 130–1
  drinking in moderation 71–72
  and the skin 130–1
algotherapy/seaweed wraps 102
allergies 144
alpha hydroxy acids (AHAs) 119
aluminium 27, 101
amber 178
amethyst 180
analgesia 82, 145
animal essences 181–5
antioxidants 124–6
appetite suppressants 54–6
arthritis 143, 145
asthma 144
astrology 148, 167–170

Bach's Flower Remedies 174–6
back pain 144, 145
bacteria, in tap water 27
balneotherapy 102
Banana Breakfast (recipe) 52
bathing 92–94
  see also showering
  bowl bathing 85

brief history of 76–7
candle bathing 92–3
Dead Sea bathing 99–100, 104
Ginger Warmer bath 94
Kneipp bathing 84–5
Revitalising Refresher bath 93–4
salt bathing 104–5
in thalassotherapy 102, 104–5
Water Detox bath 20
Batmanghelidj, F. 142
Beans and Herbs (recipe) 64–5
beauty *see* skin care
Beetroot and Tzatziki (recipe) 67
bergamot tea 73
beta-carotene 124
bicarbonates 34
birth defects 28
bloating 32, 133
blood plasma 99
blood pressure 143
blue 188, 189
'blue baby syndrome' 29
body
  illness 138–46
  moisturisers 123
  pH 139, 145
  use of water 10–12, 19, 35–9, 141
  water content 10–11, 12, 39–40,
    141
body temperature
  high 45, 79
  regulation 38

body wraps
  algotherapy/seaweed 102
  clay/deep-sea mud 104
bottled water 24–5, 31–6
  convenience of 35–6
  drinking water 31
  fizzy 31–2
  flavoured 31
  natural mineral water 32–5
  purified water 32
  spring water 32
  table water 32
bowl bathing 85
brain, water content of 10–11
breakfast 45, 51–4
Breakfast Pick-me-up (recipe) 51
bromides 100
brumisation 103

cabbage 47, 62
caffeine
  see also coffee
  diuretic effect of 43, 130–1
  effect on homeopathic remedies 173
  effect on the skin 130–1
calcium 34, 100, 125
cancer 12, 29, 130
Cancer (astrological sign) 168–9
candle bathing 92–3
canoeing 112
carbon filters 30
carbonated water 31
cell metabolism, boosters for 80
cellulite 7, 131–7
  causes of 131–7
  and convenience foods 133–4
  and fluid retention 132–3, 134
  and food intolerances 135–6
  and inactivity 136–7
  and yo-yo dieting 134–5
ceramides 120
chamomile tea 73
checklist 8
cheese 46, 48, 63, 70
Cheese and Celery Plate (recipe) 70
Chinese traditions
  face reading 38

Feng Shui 148, 156–164
chloride 34
chlorine, in tap water 27
circulation 80, 145
citrine 180
clay/deep-sea mud wraps 104
cleansers 128–9
coffee
  see also caffeine
  diuretic effect of 43
  drinking in moderation 71–2
  substitutes for 22
Coghill, Roger 164, 166
colas 43
cold treatments, in hydrotherapy 77–8,
    82–6, 87, 88
colds 145
collagen 120
colonic irrigation 88–9
colour healing 185, 187–9
computer screens 167
constipation 145
convenience foods 133–4
cooking methods 49
cooking oils 46, 48
coriander 97
Coyote (animal essence) 183
crewing 112
Crow (animal essence) 185
crudités 55
cryotherapy 103
crystal essences/spritz 176–81
  how to make 181
  types of crystal 178–80
curries 45
cystitis 145

dandelion 45
Dead Sea bathing 99–100, 104
dehydration
  effects of 11
  and fluid retention 132–3
  and illness 139, 142
  and the skin 126
  symptoms of 2, 40
'dehydration mode' 135
desserts 70–1

Detox Paella (recipe) 61
diamond 178
dieting
  see also nutrition
  yo-yo 134–5
dinners, recipes for 56–70
diuretics 43–6
  alcohol 44, 130–1
  coffee/caffeine/stimulant
     drinks 43, 130–1
  illness/recovery 45
  physical exercise 44
  sleep 44
  stimulant foods 45
  urination 45–6
diving 113–14
dolphins, swimming with 91–2
domestic water 12, 13
drinking water 21–23, 32
  how to 21–2, 44
  with meals 23, 71–2
  too much too soon 22, 23
  when to 22–3
droughts 13
drugs, in tap water 29
dry skin brushing 126
Dull, Harold 90
dyspepsia 145

earth element 159, 160
electric blankets 166
electromagnetic fields (EMFs) 148,
    151–2, 164–7, 189–90
emerald 179
emotions
  flower remedies for 174–6
  and the moon 147–8, 154
energy, flow of 160–2
Epsom salts 104, 107
essential oils
  for bathing 20
  for the skin 122–3
  use in hydrotherapy 86–7, 92–3, 96
eucalyptus 96
exfoliation 17
  Honey Body smoother 127–8
  Rice Polish 127

Simple Salt scrub 128–9
  in thalassotherapy 103

face reading, Chinese 38
Feng Shui 156–64
  five elements 158–62
  good water/negative water 162
  practitioners 158
fennel 97
fertility 153
Feta and Watermelon (recipe) 53
fever 79
filtered water 26, 29–30
  carbon filters 30
  installed water filters 30
  reverse osmosis 30, 32
fire element 159, 160
fish 46, 48, 67–70
five elements 158–62
  controlling cycle 159–60
  supporting cycle 159'
fizzy water 22, 31–2
  carbonated 32
  naturally sparkling 31–2
flavonoids 72
flavoured water 31
flotation 104, 105–8
  see also Watsu
flower remedies 174–6
fluid retention 132–3, 134
fluoride 27–8
fluorites 179
food intolerances 135–6
  see also nutrition
Fresh Fish Ceviche (recipe) 69
fresh water 21, 22
fruit 47, 48, 56, 70
fruit cordials 22
fruit juices 22, 51–52
Fruit Salad (recipe) 54
Garlic Crush (recipe) 63
Garlic and Ginger Vegetables with Goat's or
    Sheep's Cheese (recipe) 63
germs, in tap water 27
ginger tea 73
Ginger Warmer (bath) 94
ginseng tea 73

grapefruit 96
Grapeful (recipe) 52
gravity 150, 152
green 187, 188
Green Soup (recipe) 57–8
green tea 72
greens 47
Grilled Kippers and Tomatoes (recipe) 52
Grilled Pineapple and Honey (recipe) 53
Grilled Sardines (recipe) 68
Grilled Tuna with Anchovy Lattice (recipe) 70

Hahnemann, Samuel 171
hard water 28
headaches 145
healing waters 6, 8, 138–146, 148, 170–185
    animal essences 181–5
    for common ailments 142–6
    crystal essences 176–81
    flower remedies 174–6
    homeopathy 171–3
heart conditions 28, 143
heartburn 145
heat stroke 81
heat treatments, in hydrotherapy 78–81, 83, 84–6
herbal teas 22
    as appetite suppressants 55
    diuretic 45
    recommended 48, 72–4
herbicides, in tap water 29
herbs
    dietary 48
    use in hydrotherapy 96–7
holidays 149
homeopathy 171–73
Honey Body smoother (exfoliator) 127–8
Honey Nut 'Soups' (recipe) 71
hormones, and cellulite 131
Hot Grilled Cabbage (recipe) 62
humectants 120
Hummus (recipe) 55
hunger pangs 4, 54, 144
hydrotherapy 4–5, 8, 75–97
    bathing 78, 92–4

cold treatments 78, 82–6, 87, 88
colonic irrigation 88–9
defining 75
heat treatments 77–81, 83, 84–8
herbs for 97
jacuzzis 87–8
Kneipp bathing 84–5
oils for 96
saunas and steamrooms 86–7
swimming with dolphins 91–2
walking by the sea 89–90
Watsu 90–1

illness 138–46
    allergies 144
    arthritis 143, 145
    asthma 144
    back pain 144, 145
    blood pressure 143
    diuretic effect of 45
    dyspepsia/heartburn/indigestion 145
    excess weight 144
    heart conditions 143
indigestion 145
inflammation 82–3
intestines, use of water 39
Invigorator, The (shower) 95
iodine 101

Jacket Potatoes (recipe) 57
jacuzzis 87–8
juices 22, 51–2
juniper 45

kidneys, use of water 37
Kneipp bathing 84–5

labradorite 179
lapis lazuli 179
lavender essential oil 20, 96, 122
lead, in tap water 28
leftovers 56
lipids 120
liver, use of water 36–7
lunches, recipes for 56–70
lungs, use of water 38–9
lymphatic system
    boosters for 80

and cellulite 136
use of water 37–8

magnesium 34, 101, 104
magnetism 189–90
    see also electromagnetism
malachite 180
Mango Salad (recipe) 66
maté tea 73
meals
    drinking water with 23, 71
    eating little and often 48, 49–50, 56
meditation 105–6
menstrual cycle 155
metabolism, boosters for 80
metal element 159, 160
microwaves 167
mineral water, natural 32–4
minerals, in seawater 99–102
mobile phones 166
Moisturiser, The (shower) 96
moisturisers 116, 119–23
    alpha hydroxy acids 119
    for the body 123
    ceramides 120
    collagen 120
    humectants 120
    lipids 120
    natural 121–3
    retinoids and retin A 120
moon 150–6
    'blue' 156
    dark phase 153, 154–5
    effect on water 150
    'female' 155
    full 153, 153–4
    lunar cycle 152
    new 153
    waning 153, 154–5
Moon Diary 7, 147–8
Moon Mother 154
mud wraps 104
Muesli (recipe) 53
muscles
    cold treatments for 82
    heat treatments for 81
muscular spasticity 81

music 185, 189
myoneural junction 81

Native American tradition 150, 181–5
natural mineral water 32–4
naturally sparkling water 31
necrosin 82
neroli 96
nettle tea 45
New Potato Salad with Beans and Peas
    (recipe) 62
nickel 101
nitrates, in tap water 29
Nut Salad (recipe) 66
nutrition 4, 41–75
    and cellulite 133–4
    cooking methods 49
    diuretics 43–6
    drinking with food 23, 71
    foods with high-water content 4, 42
    how to eat and drink 46–9
    recipe suggestions 50–74
    recommended foods 46–8
    for the skin 123–6
nuts 48

oils
    cooking 46, 48
    essential 20, 86–7, 92–3, 96, 122–3
    for the skin 122–3
onions 47
opal 178
orange (colour) 188, 189
orange essential oil 20
Oven-baked Stuffed Vegetables (recipe) 64

pain relief 82, 145
parsley 97
Pear, Walnut and Rocket Salad with
    Roquefort (recipe) 65
peppermint tea 73
pesticides, in tap water 29
pH, of the body 139, 145
physical exercise
    diuretic effect of 44
    drinking water during 22
    watercise 5, 109–15

Pisces 168
planetary water 13
plunge pools 87
potassium 34, 101, 133–4
potatoes 46, 62
potentising 170, 171
premature ageing 129–30
pulse rate, boosters for 80
pulses 47
Pumpkin Soup (recipe) 58
purified water 32
purple 188, 189

quartz 178–9

radio alarm clocks 166
Rainbow Rice (recipe) 60
raspberry leaf tea 73
raw foods 49
recipes 50–74
   Banana Breakfast 52
   Beans and Herbs 64–5
   Beetroot and Tzatziki 67
   Breakfast Pick-me-up 51
   breakfasts 51–4
   Cheese and Celery Plate 70
   desserts 70–1
   Detox Paella 61
   Feta and Watermelon 53
   Fresh Fish Ceviche 69
   Fruit Salad 54
   Garlic Crush 63
   *Garlic and Ginger Vegetables with Goat's
     or Sheep's Cheese* 63
   Grapeful 52
   Green Soup 57–8
   Grilled Kippers and Tomatoes 52
   Grilled Pineapple and Honey 53
   Grilled Sardines 68
   *Grilled Tuna with Anchovy
     Lattice* 70
   Honey Nut 'Soups' 71
   Hot Grilled Cabbage 62
   Hummus 55
   Jacket Potatoes 57
   lunches and dinners 56–70
   Mango Salad 66

   Muesli 53
   New Potato Salad with Beans and Peas 62
   Nut Salad 66
   Oven-baked Stuffed Vegetables 64
   *Pear, Walnut and Rocket Salad with
     Roquefort* 65
   Pumpkin Soup 58
   Rainbow Rice 60
   Red Rice Salad 59
   Roast Broccoli with Tuna 67
   St Clement's 51
   Salmon and Tarragon 69
   snacks 54–6
   Steamed Fish with Ginger 68
   Stir Fried Rice 59–60
   Tomato Gazpacho 58–9
   Tuna Rice 68
   Watermelon Wake-up 52
   Wild Rice and Salsa 61–2
   Yoghurt Dips 65
recovery from illness, diuretic effect of 45
red 187, 188
Red Rice Salad (recipe) 59
relaxation 148, 185–90
resonant frequencies 185
retin A 120
retinoids 120
retinol 124
reverse osmosis 30, 32
Revitalising Refresher (bath) 93–4
rice 47, 48, 59–61
Rice Polish (exfoliator) 127
rivers, walking along 114
Roast Broccoli with Tuna (recipe) 67
rose essential oil 20
rose quartz 179
rosemary 96
rule of 12 173

sage 97
sailing 109–10
St Clement's (recipe) 51
salads 47, 59, 65–6
Salmon and Tarragon (recipe) 69
salt
   bathing 104–5
   dietary 133–4

sandalwood 96
saunas 86–7
Scorpio 169–70
sea
    see also thalassotherapy
    walking by 89–90
seasoning 48
seawater
    baths 102
    constituents of 100–102
seaweed wraps 102
sebum 118
sedentary lifestyles, and cellulite 131
selenium 101, 124
'shock effect', beneficial 82
showering 17, 94–6
    see also bathing
    The Invigorator 95
    The Moisturiser 96
Simple Salt scrub (exfoliator) 128–9
skiing 113
skin 5, 7, 116–137
    and alcohol consumption 130–1
    of the body 123–4
    and caffeine 130–1
    care routine for 116
    and cellulite 131–7
    cleansing 128–9
    composition of 117–119
    dry skin brushing 126
    moisturising 116, 119–23
    nutrition for 123–6
    oils for 122–3
    saunas and steamrooms for 86–7
    and sunbathing 129–30
    tips for 116–17
    use of water 38
skin cancer 130
sleep 44–5
smoking 39
smoothies 51–2
snacks, recipes for 54–6
snowflake obsidian (Apache tears) 180
sodalite 180
sodium 34, 101, 133
soft water 28
soups 57–8

spas 76, 84–5
spasticity 81
spices 45
spring water 32
star signs 148, 167–70
'starvation mode' 135
Steamed Fish with Ginger (recipe) 68
steaming 49
steamrooms 86–7
stimulant drinks, diuretic effect of 43
stimulant foods, diuretic effect of 45
Stir Fried Rice (recipe) 59–60
stir frying 49, 59–60
streams 114
stress 146, 186
succussion 171
sulphates 34
sulphur 101
sun 152
sunbathing 129–30
sweat lodges 149–50
swimming 110–11
    with dolphins 91–2
swimming pools 115

table water 32
tap water 25, 26–31
    cleaning 29–31
    content of 26–9
    filtration methods for 26
tarragon 97
tea 22, 72
    see also herbal teas
televisions 167
thalassotherapy 5, 7, 98–108
    algotherapy/seaweed wraps 102
    balneotherapy 102
    baths 102, 104–5
    body/exfoliating scrubs 103
    brumisation 103
    buoyancy 100, 104
    clay/deep-sea mud wraps 104
    cryotherapy 103
    Dead Sea bathing 104
    flotation 104, 105–8
    salt bathing 104–5
    seawater minerals 99–102

thiamine 125
thirst, misinterpretation as hunger 4, 54, 144
tides 150, 152
tiger's eye 178
tisanes 55, 72–3
Tomato Gazpacho (recipe) 58–9
tomatoes 47, 58–9
tooth decay, prevention 27–8
tourmaline 180
toxins, elimination 35–9, 41–2, 88–9
Tuna Rice (recipe) 68
turquoise 180

urination 45–6
UVA/UVB rays 130

vasoconstriction 82, 84
vasodilation 79–80, 84
vegetables 47, 48
vertebral discs 144
vitamin A 124
vitamin C 124
vitamin D 124–5, 125
vitamin E 125

walking
   along rivers 114
   by the sea 89–90
water 4, 10–40
   appreciation of 7, 16–20
   body's use of 10–11, 13, 20, 35–9, 141
   chemical composition of 14–15, 162
   cleansing effect of 39–40
   defining 14–16
   domestic use of 12, 13
   drinking 21–23, 32, 44, 71
   effect of the moon on 150–2
   electrical charge of 14–15
   facts 10–12
   in Feng Shui 156–8, 162–4
   fresh 21, 22
   functions of 15–16, 17–20
   history of 190–1
   holidays near 149–50
   magnetising 189–90
   memory of 171–3
   physical properties of 14
   planetary 13
   recommended amounts 49
   for the skin 125–6
   types of 23–36
water analysis 26
water authorities 26, 28
Water Detox Bath 20
water medicine *see* healing water
water retention 132–3, 134
water-loss *see* diuretics
watercise 5, 109–15
   canoeing 112
   diving 113–14
   sailing 111–12
   skiing 113
   swimming 110–11
   swimming pools 115
   travelling to waterfalls 114
   walking along rivers 114
   windsurfing 112–13
waterfalls 114
Watermelon Wake–up (recipe) 52
Watsu 90–1
wealth 156–64
weight
   excess 144
   loss 4
white 188
Wild Rice and Salsa (recipe) 61–2
windsurfing 112–13
wood element 159, 160
wraps
   algotherapy/seaweed 102
   clay/deep-sea mud 104
wrinkles 118

yellow 187, 188
yin & yang 155, 160
ylang ylang essential oil 20
yo-yo dieting 134–5
yoghurt 46, 54, 65
Yoghurt Dips (recipe) 65

zinc 101, 125

48 Hour Detox

Jane Scrivner

Do your mind and body feel sluggish and dull?

Would you like to feel like a million dollars at very little expense?

Do you have 48 hours to transport yourself to an oasis of calm and cleansing?

Do you want your next weekend to feel like a two-week holiday?

Have you got just two days to discover the new you?

In *48 Hour Detox* best-selling author Jane Scrivner provides a two-day transformation plan to revitalise your mind, body and spirit. She gives you a well-balanced, easy-to-follow programme that you can undertake over a weekend or on holiday. There is even guidance on detoxing to help you recover during illness or convalescence.

- Provides complete lists for foods, supplements and equipment needed
- Details a fun programme of exercise, diet and relaxation for the full two-day period
- Provides easy-to-follow recipes for relaxing aromatherapy baths
- Reveals step-by-step guidelines for massage therapies
- Details a step-by-step yoga stretch session
- Provides quick and easy recipes for each meal of the two-day programme
- Provides guided meditations to help you relax and unwind
- Details how to create your own healing home spa

£4.99

TOTAL DETOX

6 ways to revitalise your life

Jane Scrivner

The be-all-and-end-all Detox bestseller in a handy pocket-size format.

Do you want to clear your mind and re-energise your body?

Are you stressed out by 21st-century living?

Total Detox is the key to looking good, feeling great and living your life to the full. Jane Scrivner, co-founder of The British School of Complementary Therapy and bestselling author of *Detox Yourself*, has created 6 outstanding detox programmes. Each is designed to suit a specific need, from the 30-Day Ultimate Detox to the Relationship Detox. Whatever the situation and whatever your lifestyle, this book provides all you'll ever need to feel healthy, happy and completely invigorated.

£6.99

LaStone Therapy

Jane Scrivner

In *LaStone Therapy*, bestselling Detox author Jane Scrivner introduces you to an exciting new form of bodywork. LaStone massage therapy is a modern technique drawing on ancient Native American traditions and using heated and cooled stones on the body. Created in 1993 in Arizona, and already the fastest-growing bodywork therapy in the US, LaStone delivers on every level: body, mind and spirit; physically, emotionally and energetically. Written with the full co-operation of, and in consultation with, the creator of LaStone therapy – under whom Jane herself was trained – this book

- Explains what this treatment is, where it came from and what it does
- Shows how even just one treatment will make you feel fabulous
- Describes exactly how LaStone gets deeper, more quickly, and lasts much, much longer than conventional massage
- Details the chemistry of thermotherapy – the alternating therapeutic application of hot and cold temperatures – and how it can achieve far more than conventional bodywork techniques
- Reveals how LaStone can prolong the working life of the therapist while simultaneously improving the health of the client
- Provides a comprehensive resources list so that you can experience LaStone – or even train as a therapist – yourself

£8.99

If you have enjoyed reading this book, you may be interested in other health titles published by Piatkus.
You can order them online at www.piatkus.co.uk or call 01476 541080.

10 Days to Better Health
Nic Rowley and Kirsten Hartvig
£6.99

100 Ways to Live to be 100
Dr Roger Henderson
£7.99

The 30-Day Fatburner Diet
Patrick Holford
£6.99

Acupressure
Michael Reed Gach
£14.99

The Alternative Pregnancy Handbook
Dr Tanvir Jamil and Karen Evenett
£10.99

Alzheimer's Disease
Frena Gray-Davidson
£9.99

Balancing Hormones Naturally
Kate Neil and Patrick Holford
£5.99

Be Your Own Best Friend
Louis Proto
£6.99

Beat Cellulite Forever
Dr James Fleming
£6.99

Beat Stress And Fatigue
Patrick Holford
£5.99

The Bodycode Diet and Fitness Programme
Jay Cooper with Kathryn Lance
£6.99

Boost Your Child's Immune System
Lucy Burney
£6.99

Boost Your Immune System
Jennifer Meek and Patrick Holford
£5.99

The Change Before The Change
Dr Laura E Corio & Linda G Kahn
£16.99

The Complete Book of Ayurvedic Home Remedies
Vasant Lad
£13.99

The Complete Book of Food Combining
Kathryn Marsden
£12.99

Daniele Ryman's Aromatherapy Bible
Daniele Ryman
£12.99

Detox Your Life
Jane Scrivner
£6.99

Detox Your Mind
Jane Scrivner
£6.99

Detox Yourself
Jane Scrivner
£6.99

Dr Gillian McKeith's Living Food for Health
Gillian McKeith
£7.99

The Eat To Live Diet
Joel Fuhrman
£6.99

Endless Energy
Fiona Agombar
£6.99

Energy Medicine
Donna Eden
£14.99

Fibromyalgia
Dr Don L. Goldenberg
£10.99

Fight Fat After Forty
Dr Pamela Peeke
£7.99

Fitness For the Over 60s
Susie Dinan and Dr Craig Sharp
£10.99

Good Gut Healing
Kathryn Marsden
£10.99

The H Factor
Patrick Holford & Dr James Braly
£8.99

The Healing Journey
Matthew Manning
£14.99

Improve Your Digestion
Patrick Holford
£5.99

Introduction to Reiki
Penelope Quest
£6.99

LaStone Therapy
Jane Scrivner
£8.99

The Lazy Girl's Guide to a Fabulous Body
Anita Naik
£7.99

The Lazy Girl's Guide to Beauty
Anita Naik
£7.99

The Lazy Girl's Guide To Good Health
Anita Naik
£7.99

The Little Book Of Detox
Jane Scrivner
£2.99

The Little Book of Optimum Nutrition
Patrick Holford
£2.50

The Live-Longer Diet
Sally Beare
£9.99

Look 10 Years Younger
Margareta Loughran
£10.99

Lower Your Blood Pressure in 8 Weeks
Dr Stephen T Sinatra
£12.99

Macrobiotics
Jon Sandifer
£9.99

The Metabolic Anti-Ageing Plan
Stephen Cherniske MSc
£12.99

Natural Healing
Chrissie Wildwood
£10.99

Natural Health Handbook for Women
Marilyn Glenville
£20.00

Natural Healthcare for Children
Karen Sullivan
£14.99

Natural Highs
Patrick Holford
£14.99

Natural Highs – Chill
Patrick Holford and Hyla Cass
£5.99

Natural Highs – Energy
Patrick Holford and Hyla Cass
£5.99

Natural Solutions to Infertility
Marilyn Glenville
£12.99

Natural Solutions To PMS
Marilyn Glenville
£10.99

The Nutritional Health Handbook for Women
Marilyn Glenville
£16.99

The Optimum Nutrition Bible
Patrick Holford
£12.99

Optimum Nutrition for the Mind
Patrick Holford
£12.99

Organic Living in 10 Simple Lessons
Karen Sullivan
£12.99

Perfect Skin
Amanda Cochrane
£9.99

The Period Book
Karen Gravelle and Jennifer Gravelle
£7.50

Qigong for Harmony and Relaxation
Michael Tse
£12.99

The Quick-Fix Hangover Detox
Jane Scrivner
£4.99

The Reflexology Handbook
Laura Norman
£16.99

Reiki For Life
Penelope Quest
£12.99

Say No To Arthritis
Patrick Holford
£8.99

Say No To Cancer
Patrick Holford
£5.99

Say No to Heart Disease
Patrick Holford
£5.99

Self Healing
Louis Proto
£6.99

Six Week Herbal Detox Plan
Peter Conway
£9.99

Six Weeks To Superhealth
Patrick Holford
£8.99

Solve Your Skin Problems
Natalie Savona and Patrick Holford
£5.99

The Stay Young Detox
Jane Scrivner
£6.99

Strong Women, Strong Bones
Miriam E Nelson
£12.99

Sue Kreitzman's Low Fat Lifeplan
Sue Kreitzman
£15.99

Supermodels' Beauty Secrets
Victoria Nixon
£7.99

Supplements for Superhealth
Patrick Holford
£5.99

The Tai Chi Manual
Robert Parry
£12.95

Ten Days to Better Health
Nic Rowley and Kirsten Hartvig
£8.99

Total Detox
Jane Scrivner
£6.99

Tree Medicine
Peter Conway
£14.99

Understanding Hypnosis
Dr Brian Roet
£10.99

Uplift
Barbara Delinsky
£7.99

The V Book
Dr Elizabeth Stewart
£14.99

Vertical Reflexology
Lynne Booth
£12.99

Vertical Reflexology For Hands
Lynne Booth
£12.99

Vibrational Medicine for the 21st Century
Richard Gerber
£16.99

Warriors
Robert Paterson
£9.99

The Waterfall Diet
Linda Lazarides
£6.99

Wing Chun
Grandmaster Ip Chun and Michael Tse
£12.99

The Wisdom of Menopause
Christiane Northrup
£18.99

Women's Bodies, Women's Wisdom
Christiane Northrup
£18.99

You Are What You Eat
Kirsten Hartvig ND and Dr Nic Rowley
£7.99

Your Body Speaks Your Mind
Debbie Shapiro
£11.99

Your Heart and You
Elizabeth Wilde McCormick and Dr Leisa Freeman
£9.99